Self-Therapy for the Stutterer

REVISED EDITION

Self-Therapy for the

Stutterer

–Revised Edition

Malcolm Fraser, Director
SPEECH FOUNDATION OF AMERICA

Publication No. 13, Revised Edition

Published by

Speech Foundation of America
152 Lombardy Road
Memphis, Tennessee 38111

Library of Congress Number 79-91588
ISBN 0-933388-14-4 (Hardbound)

Additional copies of this book $7.50

The Speech Foundation of America is a non-profit
charitable organization dedicated to the prevention and treatment of stuttering.

*Dedicated to all
who seek relief from the burden
of stuttering.*

To the Reader

There are always some stutterers who are unable to get professional help and others who do not seem to be able to profit from it. There are some who prefer to be their own therapists. In this book, Malcolm Fraser, Director of the Speech Foundation of America, has attempted to provide some guidance for those who must help themselves. Knowing well from his own experience as a stutterer the difficulties of self therapy, he outlines a series of objectives and challenges that should serve as a map for the person who is utterly lost in the dismal swamp of stuttering and desperately wants to find a way out.

CHARLES VAN RIPER

Distinguished Professor Emeritus and formerly Head, Department of Speech Pathology and Audiology, Western Michigan University

All the quotations and footnotes in this book have been taken from the writings of speech pathologists and medical doctors, all of whom have been stutterers themselves. They know your problems from experience. They represent a most distinguished array of authority and prestige in the field of stuttering. You will find their names listed in the appendix.

On Self-Therapy

If you are like most of the million and a half stutterers
in this country, clinical treatment will not be available
to you. Whatever you do you'll have to be pretty much
on your own with what ideas and sources you can use.

(Sheehan)

The first thing you must do is to admit to yourself
that you need to change, that you really want to do
something about the way you presently talk. This is
tough but your commitment must be total; not even a
small part of you must hold back. Don't dwell longingly
on your fluency in the magical belief that some day your
speech blocks will disappear. There is no magic potion,
no pink pill that will cure stuttering.

Don't sit around waiting for the right time for an inspiration to come to you—*you must go to it.* You must
see that the old solutions, the things you have done to
help yourself over the years simply do not work. Ruts
wear deep though, and you will find it difficult to change.
Even though the way you presently talk is not particularly pleasant, it is familiar. It is the unknown from
which we shrink.

You must be willing to endure temporary discomfort,
perhaps even agony for the long range improvement you
desire. No one is promising you a rose garden. Why not
take the time and effort now for a lifetime of freedom
from your tangled tongue? How can you do this? You
break down the global problem of stuttering into its
smaller parts and then solve them one at a time. It's
simple. No one said it was easy. Shall we begin?

(Emerick)

A valuable precondition for a successful therapy is
the deep inner conviction of the stutterer in the
curability of his disorder, combined with a fighting spirit
and a readiness to undergo hardships and deprivations
if needed—hopelessness, pessimism and passivity being
the deadliest foes to self-improvement.

(Freund)

On This Approach to Self-Therapy

This book is written to and for the many adult stutterers in this country[1]—and is addressed in the second person to describe what the stutterer can and should do to control his stuttering. We state confidently that as a stutterer you do not need to surrender helplessly to your speech difficulty because you can change the way you talk. You can learn to communicate with ease rather than with effort. There is no quick and easy way to tackle the problem but with the right approach self-therapy can be effective.

Experience has probably taught you to be skeptical about any plan which claims to offer a solution to your stuttering problem. You may have tried different ideas and been disappointingly disillusioned in the past. This book promises no quick magical cure and makes no false claims. It describes what you can and should do to overcome your difficulty.

It offers a logical practical program of therapy for the stutterer based on methods and procedures that have been used successfully in certain university and other speech clinics. This approach to therapy has been shown to get results. If there were an easier or better way of learning to control stuttering we would recommend it.

---

[1]Almost one percent of the population of this country manifest some acute form of stammering speech, which places them under a great economic and social handicap. This can be corrected if given the proper training. (Martin) (Note: Stammering and stuttering are the same.)

We start with two assumptions. One is that you have no physical defect or impairment of your speech mechanism. If you can talk without stuttering when you are alone or when not being heard or observed by others, it would be a fair assumption that you have no physical or organic defect causing your trouble.[1, 2, 3] Actually all stutterers have periods of fluency.

The other assumption is that you are not in position to avail yourself of the services of a speech pathologist trained to help you work on your problem in the manner described in this book and that, as a result you need to be your own therapist. Certainly you need guidance, but stuttering therapy is largely a do-it-yourself project anyway.[4, 5, 6, 7]

---

[1]We know that in stuttering there is nothing organically wrong with the organs of speech. Under certain favorable conditions every stutterer can speak without a sign of hesitation. This would be impossible if any physiological defect existed. (Wedberg)

[2]There is no physical reason why you can't learn to speak more easily and fluently than you do now. (Johnson)

[3]There is nothing wrong inside your body that will stop you from talking. You have the same speaking equipment as anybody else. You have the ability to talk normally. (D. Williams)

[4]No one but myself improved my speech. Others have helped me by providing information, giving emotional support, identifying bias, etc. but the dirty work of therapy is, and always has been, my responsibility. (Boehmler)

[5]Don't ever forget that even if you went to the most knowledgeable expert in the country, the correction of stuttering is a do-it-yourself project. Stuttering is your problem. The expert can tell you what to do and how to do it, but you are the one who has to do it. You are the only person on earth who can correct your stuttering. (Starbuck)

[6]The stutterer must conquer his own problem - no one else can do the job for him. (VanRiper)

[7]Needless to say, each stutterer must from the beginning of therapy accept the responsibility for his problem. This implies self-therapy which is essential. (Stromsta)

If you are sincerely interested in working on your speech you will need to have a strong motivation to overcome your difficulty and a sincere determination to follow through on the suggested procedures and assignments. Otherwise there is no use in trying this approach to self-therapy. It will not be easy, but it can be done.

Obviously there is no way to promise success in this or any other program since no sure 'cure' for stuttering has yet been discovered, in spite of what you may have read. However, we believe that if you follow the suggestions and carry out the procedures outlined in this book, you should be able to control your stuttering and speak easily and without abnormality. Others have conquered their stuttering and you can too. But the best way for you to judge the effectiveness of any therapy program is to try it out and let the results speak for themselves.[1]

In starting this approach to therapy it might be well to point out that there is a great amount of difference among stutterers. Some cases are mild and others severe. And the frequency and severity of your stuttering will usually vary from time to time and from one situation to another.

Also there are many ways of stuttering. No two people stutter alike as every stutterer has developed his own particular pattern of stuttering.[2] Your reactions may be different from others and accordingly we ask you to bear with us when you read about blocking diffi-

---

[1]Based on your understanding choose the most appropriate therapy program you can, and work at the program with more consistency, devotion and energy than any other task you've ever tackled. As success is obtained, maintain it with equal vigor. (Boehmler)

[2]The old saying that no two stutterers are alike is undoubtedly true. (Luper)

culties which you do not encounter yourself but which may represent a problem to other stutterers.

Equipment Desirable. For use in your work and study in this program it would help to have three items available. One is a reasonably large mirror (at least 15" x 18") which can be moved around unless it is now situated where you can observe yourself closely when talking on the telephone. And it would be desirable if you could obtain the use of a small portable dictating machine or tape recorder[1,2] of a size not much bigger than your hand which you can carry around with you to record your speech. It can be purchased at a fairly reasonable price. And you should also have on hand a small memorandum notebook.

Original Cause of Your Stuttering

One general comment is worth mentioning and should be of interest. There is no reason to be concerned about the original cause of your stuttering. Many theories have been advanced to explain its cause and nature, but none of them have been proven or seem provable. It may have resulted from an interaction of environmental and hereditary factors.

Whatever the cause, it is unlikely that it is still operating upon you or that it can be corrected at this late date. Therefore we do not believe that the original cause of your stuttering has or should have any bearing on or

---

[1] A tape recorder will prove a good investment for the stammerer. (Bluemel)

[2] By using a tape recorder you tend to learn faster that your stuttering is, indeed, your own doing, and the changes you can make in what you do are very substantial. (Johnson)

affect the therapy process.[1] You need to be concerned about what you are doing now that perpetuates and maintains your difficulty.

There is no reason for you to spend the rest of your life stuttering helplessly and making yourself miserable. Others have prevailed and so can you.

In case you are not familiar with the meanings of some of the words used in stuttering therapy, you will find a glossary in the back of this book where definitions are given of terms and expressions used in the treatment of stuttering including many not found in this book. Read them for your general education in speech pathology.

[1]Many stutterers have mistakenly believed that if only the "cause" could be found, a fast cure would result. (Murray)

Reminder—the footnotes in this book were taken from the writings of men and women who have known what you are up against since they have all been stutterers themselves. Nearly all of these speech pathologists have earned degrees as doctors of philosophy or medicine and distinguished themselves in the field of stuttering. Their names and titles are listed in the appendix.

The Premise, the Program and Determination

The ideas expressed in this book are based on the premise that stuttering is not a symptom of something but is a behavior that can be modified.[1] This means that you can learn to control your difficulty, partly through modifying your feelings and attitudes about stuttering, and partly through modifying the irregular behaviors associated with your stuttering blocks.[2, 3, 4]

This will include analyzing your stuttering behavior, eliminating what you do which is unnecessary or abnormal, taking positive action to control your blocks, and reducing your emotional reactions by disciplining yourself to face your fears and become less sensitive about

---

[1]The basic fact revealed by these laboratory and clinical studies was that the behavior called stuttering is extremely modifiable. It is possible for a speaker to change drastically the things he does that he calls his stuttering. (Johnson)

[2]Your fundamental task is twofold; alter your speech behavior, and bring about positive changes in your self-perception and feelings. (Murray)

[3]During the process of therapy he (the stutterer) should learn by experience that he can change his speaking behavior and that he can change his emotional reactions, both to the way he talks and toward his listeners and himself. (D. Williams)

[4]Basically there are two principal features of his behavior that the stutterer can alter. One is the speech behavior itself and the other is his attitude toward speaking and stuttering in particular. These two aspects are related: one of the ways change of attitude is brought about is by helping the stutterer to experience an ability to modify his speech, and one way in which speech is changed is through the reduction of fear which accompanies a different way of thinking about the problem. (Gregory)

your disorder.[1, 2] The basic principle is that stuttering is something you are doing and you can learn to change what you are doing.[3]

About the Program

Since it is important for you to understand the overall therapy plan, we explain briefly how this program works. First you are asked to comply with nine commonsense helpful recommendations or ground rules that will improve your speech.

In complying with these rewarding ground rules you will be concentrating on reducing the severity and abnormality of your stutterings. When this reduction occurs the number of your stutterings will also decline. It is essential that you do your best to comply with these ground rules. They will lay the groundwork and help you make progress.

In the next phase you will investigate your stuttering behavior and work on eliminating any undesirable or unattractive behaviors you may have developed, associated with your stuttering, which are not directly involved in the production of speech. These include eliminating any restraining or frustrating habits you may have acquired as a result of your efforts to hide, avoid or disguise your stuttering.

---

[1]Somehow you must learn to desensitize yourself to the reactions of others and refuse to let people's actual or imagined responses to your stuttering continue to affect your mental health or peace of mind. (Adler)

[2]One of the most important phases of the treatment of the adult stutterer is that which attempts to change the shame and embarrassment that are associated with the act of stuttering. (VanRiper)

[3]Stuttering consists mainly of learned behavior. This behavior can be unlearned. (Murray)

The last phase calls for you first to make a detailed study of what is happening with your speech muscles when you stutter. This is important because you need to find out exactly what you are doing incorrectly in order to correct it.[1] Then you will be instructed how to cope with these errors by using post-block, in-block or pre-block corrections to modify or reverse such faulty speech muscle behavior. These corrections are designed to help you move easily and smoothly through feared words in a predetermined manner so you will develop a feeling of control.

When you find that you can comply with the ground rules, you will have made real progress in controlling your speech. To make further progress you are asked to work on each of the other steps in order as they are described in this book.

Some of the ground rules or steps will mean more to you and affect your stuttering more than others, because they will hit your weak points where you need the most help. As a result you may find that attaining the goal of some ground rule or step will contribute more to progress in your case than some of the others. Unfortunately there is no way for us to know your particular weaknesses, so we must ask that you follow the program as outlined.

The length of time needed to accomplish the objective of each rule or step will vary considerably according to the severity of your case, and your resolution in work-

---

[1]You've got to examine and analyze the act of speaking to see what errors you're making. You must be making mistakes somewhere or you would be speaking fluently. What are you doing that makes your speech come out as stuttering? (Starbuck)

ing on the assignments. It is possible that the time required to reach some desired goal can be measured in days, but for some stutterers it may take a long time to bring under control some stubborn or seemingly uncontrollable practice or habit.[1, 2]

Even if your stuttering is mild you should move through each phase of the program as outlined.[3] And when you tackle the assignments you should feel satisfied that you have reasonably achieved the goal or purpose of each ground rule or step before proceeding to the next one. By doing this you will know exactly where you stand and what progress you are making. To repeat—the program should be performed and completed step-by-step.

About Your Determination

For therapy to be a success it will take a lot of determination on your part to follow through on the various assignments.[4] It will be necessary for you to be brave since you will need to confront[5] your stuttering head-on

---

[1]The adult stutterer enters therapy . . . the first thing he must understand is that stuttering as it now exists was acquired over a period of time, and that change is a process which will be gradual - not sudden. (Gregory)

[2]But you say you want to stop stuttering. Sure! But first you need to break up the habit pattern that you have built up over the years and this cannot be done instantly. (Emerick)

[3]Therefore we must proceed up a long ladder of sub-goals, each of which takes you closer to the conquest of your speech defect. (VanRiper)

[4]You appreciate most in life those things you do for yourself. Getting over stuttering takes tremendous self-discipline and desire. (Aten)

[5]Although it is a tough row to hoe at first, there is nothing as therapeutic as self confrontation. (Rainey)

and undertake conversational experiences which may cause you embarrassment. Nevertheless, this will serve to reduce the very sensitivity that makes your stuttering worse. Becoming less sensitive to your difficulty will make it easier for you to retain sufficient presence of mind to carry through on the recommended procedures.

Now if you do not wish to go on with therapy, there are, or you can find plenty of reasons why you should not do so. Such as, for example—it's too much work and trouble—stuttering can't be cured—maybe I can find an easier approach—there is no guarantee it will work —I only stutter at times under certain circumstances —it will be too embarrassing—etc. These alibis are fine. They are only mentioned to give you the excuse you may need.

Still, as a stutterer, you need to find ways and means for having a richer life through more fluent speech.[1] You need to feel better about yourself as a person. You want to speak freely. But to do this you will need to make changes in your way of talking and in yourself that can put you in control and make you master of your speech.

We say that you can and that the pay-off is far greater than the cost. But it will take a lot of determina-

---

[1] I still remember vividly what a severe stutterer and how tangled emotionally I once was. When I see any stutterer I remember my own unfavorable prognosis, my own weakness, my lack of hope, and when I do, I find in the case before me strengths and potentials which I did not have. If I could do what I have done, then surely this person could do as much. This is a very real faith, and I suspect it has played a large part in any success I have had as a clinician. (VanRiper)

tion on your part.[1] Stuttering is a stubborn handicap and it will not give up easily.[2] Therapy is a challenge.[3] What is your alternative?

---

[1]Leonard, a stutterer, would try anything, although never in a reckless or foolhardy fashion. He possessed both discernment enough to see what needed to be done and guts enough to do it - a happy combination for a stutterer. He had kind of a stubbornness or dogged persistence that he was able to turn into an asset. (Sheehan)

[2]Stuttering is a tough opponent. It never gives up. You've got to keep knocking it down to stay in command. (Starbuck)

[3]Men who have achieved in this world have been guided by inspiration, by vision, by faith in themselves and by faith in the unknown. (Wedberg)

Your Feelings and Emotions

Stuttering is no simple speech impediment. It is instead a complicated disorder with both emotional and psychological aspects. To illustrate the latter, the statement can be made that stuttering is largely what the stutterer does trying not to stutter.[1] In other words it is an incredible trick which you play on yourself.

What happens is that you want to stop stuttering so badly that you try to force trouble-free speech.[2] And the more you force the more tension and trouble you have. Unfortunately, the mechanism of speech is so delicately balanced and enormously complicated that it can not be consciously controlled. So, in trying to stop stuttering, you unwittingly make it worse.

Your stuttering affects you emotionally, since being a stutterer can be rough. You may think it makes you look undignified, ineffectual and foolish and so you probably have become extremely sensitive about your difficulty.

The experience of being blocked, of not being able to say what you want to say without stuttering can be terribly frustrating.[3] As a result under some circumstances you may become so embarrassed and humiliated that you suffer miserably from feelings of helplessness, shame,

---

[1] In other words stuttering is what you do trying not to stutter again. (Johnson)

[2] The stutterer attempts to force the articulation of his words and speaking now becomes a muscular rather than a mental process. (Bluemel)

[3] Fluency is a fair-weather friend that deserts the stutterer when he needs it most. (Sheehan)

inferiority, depression, guilt and even self-hatred.[1]

These emotions may generate so much fear and anxiety that it affects your attitude toward others and your life in general.[2,3] Like the tail that wags the dog, stuttering can alter your personality structure. But if you can be toughened to it, and if you learn that you do not have to panic when stuttering threatens or is experienced, progress will come more swiftly.

Your stuttering fears can be of words or sounds, or of some persons, of certain situations, of the telephone, etc. When you have little fear you have little tension and probably don't have much difficulty. When your fear is strong you have a lot of tension and you stutter more frequently and severely. Sometimes this fear can be so strong as to drive you frantic and almost paralyze thought and action.

Fear or anxiety prevents you from entering situations and experiences that you would otherwise enjoy. This causes more frustration, and the more frustrated you become, the more you are likely to stutter. So your stuttering is usually in proportion to the amount of fear and tension you have.[4]

---

[1]Talking was a highly emotional experience which gave me a feeling of helplessness, failure and defeat. (Freund)

[2]The stutterer develops emotional reactions which permeate his very soul, affect his will and upset his mind. (Martin)

[3]The stutterer feels at most times apart and different from others in his society. He feels that although others also have difficulties in life, they can cope with them and live much more easily with their problems. He feels more permanently crippled than others because of the fact that he cannot hide or conceal his speech difficulty, and therefore, he is the constant target of their embarrassment, ridicule and disapproval. (Barbara)

[4]The more one stutters, the more he fears certain words and situations. The more he fears the more he stutters. The more he stutters the harder he struggles. The more he struggles, the more penalties he receives, and the greater becomes his fear. (VanRiper)

Tension and Relaxation

Since fear and its resulting tension are your worst enemies their reduction must be a major goal of therapy. Tension, generated by fear, plays a most important part in activating your stuttering and is probably the immediate triggering cause of your difficulty.[1] If you had little tension you probably wouldn't stutter or at least you would stutter much more easily.

It has been suggested that hypnotism might help. It sure would be marvelous if we could reduce or eliminate your tension by giving you some sort of hypnotic treatment but unfortunately it has not been shown that hypnosis has any permanent effect.[2]

In an effort to effect relaxation many stutterers have experimented with the consumption of liquor or getting slightly intoxicated. Although this is usually conducive to lessening tension and in most cases to less stuttering, its effect can only be temporary and so obviously it can not be recommended.[3]

---

[1]Stuttering results when the speaker is unable to cope with excess muscular tension in the speech mechanism. (Luper)

[2]Many of you have heard about the wonders of hypnosis and may look to this technique to provide a quick answer. Rest assured that this has been tried throughout the years, but almost invariably with only temporary and fleeting success. (Murray)

[3]One of my patients was a city official who made a practice of taking whisky before giving his weekly report to the City Council. Soon his alcoholism became a more serious problem than his stammering, and he was hospitalized for this condition. (Bluemel)

Nor, unfortunately, are there any drugs which can be recommended.[1, 2] Tranquilizers do not do the job.[3]

There also exists the hope or possibility that relaxation exercises would help to reduce tension. A lot of research has gone into studying this subject and they may be helpful in some cases. It sure would be great if one could practice some relaxation procedures which would reduce or eliminate tension and at the same time retain their effectiveness.

General relaxation procedures can frequently produce fluency, but most unfortunately it has been found that usually they have little or no carry-over effect. Many stutterers have spent thousands of hours trying them out and hoping that their effect would carry-over to their time of need, but the results have not proved satisfactory.

This does not mean that relaxation measures are discouraged since learning to relax will always benefit your general health and well-being. However, they are not indicated as a solution to your speech problem.[4] Still the fundamental principle would hold that the more relaxed and calm you are the less stuttering you will do. That's one reason you are asked to stutter easily.

---

[1]Drug treatment is strictly contraindicated. (Brown)

[2]How wonderful it would be if we could toss a pill down the throat of a stutterer and hear no more stuttering. Unfortunately we have no such panacea. (Adler)

[3]There are modern sedatives which diminish tension without inducing sleep. They may be used in an emergency but should not be relied upon to relieve a continued condition such as stammering. (Bluemel)

[4]Relaxation has sometimes been described as a method in and of itself for the treatment of stuttering. I do not believe, however, that relaxation procedures have much permanent value unless they are part of a more inclusive therapeutic process. (Gregory)

If you can locate the place where there is the most tension, it is possible that you can learn to relax those muscles during speech. And there may be certain differential muscle relaxation exercises which can be helpful under certain circumstances.

These would involve just the muscles you use to control your lips, your tongue, your mouth, your breath and to some extent the vocal cords in your throat. Later these will have limited use in the last three steps of this program.

Distractions

If there were some way you could distract your mind from thoughts of fear, so you didn't think about it, possibly you wouldn't have any trouble. If you could forget you were a stutterer you probably wouldn't stutter, but we don't know how you could develop such a "forgettery."

Anything that distracts your mind from fear or takes your mind off the threat of stuttering usually will give you temporary relief. This is the main reason why stutterers are sometimes misled by tricky procedures such as talking with sing-song inflection, or with rate control metronone timing, or talking while tapping a finger, swinging an arm, or stamping a foot etc. These and many other odd ways of talking may produce temporary fluency.

Just thinking about how to use them when you anticipate trouble, shifts your attention and temporarily blots out thoughts of fear but does not result in any permanent reduction of fear or stuttering. Strange as it may seem almost any new or bizarre technique[1, 2] may help a stutterer—at least until the novelty wears off—if he has confidence in its effectiveness and is susceptible to suggestion.

Since fear and tension are your worst enemies,[3] training in desensitization will help get rid of them. But to combat fear it will be necessary for you to torpedo a lot of your shame and sensitivity and build confidence in your ability to control your speech so that you can move smoothly through your blocks. This can be done by substituting easier ways of stuttering for your abnormal and frustrating habits. As we said before stuttering is something you are doing and you can learn to change what you are doing.

If you have made up your mind that you will work hard to overcome your difficulty by using this approach to therapy, give yourself a strong dose of will-power, have confidence in your ability to make progress and start out by doing your best to conform with the ground rules as outlined in the next chapter.

---

[1]One of the tricky features of undertaking therapy with stutterers is that anything in the way of technique to bring about immediate fluency is likely to work at least temporarily. (Sheehan)

[2]Witchcraft, the surgeon's knife, appliances for the tongue, drugs, hypnotism, psychoanalysis, arm swinging and a host of other devices and methods have been employed and a few 'cures' seem to be obtained by any method, no matter how grotesque. (VanRiper)

[3]Many stutterers learn that their greatest enemies are fear and tension. (Aten)

The Ground Rules

Adopting Rewarding Habits

In working this self-therapy program, you are asked to follow certain basic fundamental practices which we list below. These are common sense principles which by themselves will help you communicate more easily with less strain and stress. Don't just read them over. Make a sincere effort to conform to these ground rules to the best of your ability.

Remember you are your own therapist, and there is no one to supervise you if you don't follow through. Perfect compliance may not be possible and is not necessarily expected, but results are what you want and need. If you follow these recommendations the severity and frequency of your stuttering will be reduced. Here they are —there are nine of them.

(1) **Try to make a habit of talking slowly and deliberately** whether you stutter or not. It is always better to go too slow than too fast.[1] It is easier to control a slow turtle than a fast rabbit. So slow down! It will help you to speak in a more leisurely, deliberate manner if you break up your sentences into short phrases, grouping your words.

Adopting the habit of speaking slowly and deliberately may feel unnatural at first, but as you adjust to that manner of talking you will enjoy it. However, in following this recommendation, be careful and do not talk at any measured pace with rate control or timing movements in an artificial way. But say what you have to say slowly and deliberately.

---

[1]Talk slow and deliberately. (Agnello)

33

(2) **Learn to stutter easily and openly.**[1] There is nothing to be gained by struggling. The more you force, the worse your stuttering will be. Quit fighting yourself[2] —you are bound to lose.

Basically, you need to accept your problem and to cope with it without shame and embarrassment and learn to stutter without struggle and avoidance. If you comply with this one ground rule, your shame and embarrassment will diminish, your severity will lessen, and the number of your stutterings will decrease. There is a big payoff in terms of less fear and less trouble if you can just learn to stutter easily and openly.[3, 4, 5]

(3) At the moment of stuttering **try to stutter as slowly as you can.** Don't just speak slowly—stutter slowly.[6] This will be beneficial generally and also help you to learn what you are doing wrong when you stutter so that you can learn to change and control it.

(4) Try to make a habit of **speaking in a strong firm voice.** Of course you need to talk slowly and easily, but your voice should definitely not sound weak or spineless.[7] Speak up!

---

[1]Your immediate goal should be to allow yourself to stutter openly and without tension and struggle. (Murray)

[2]You do not become fluent by fighting desperately to be fluent. (J. D. Williams)

[3]Many stutterers have learned as I have learned that it is possible to stutter easily with little struggle and tension. (Sheehan)

[4]I talked (at age 35) under the illusion that speech sounds are difficult and that an enormous amount of force was necessary to overcome my self-created obstacles . . . To the stutterer, unfortunately, the use of force only compounds his difficulty. (Freund)

[5]Try to stutter more openly, more easily. (Emerick)

[6]Stutter slowly and deliberately. (Agnello)

[7]Keep going forward slowly but positively. (J. D. Williams)

(5) **Try to talk with expression and melody in your voice** without sounding affected or artificial. Avoid talking in a monotone. It is better to speak with accent in a melodius manner with a full quality voice while putting stress on the vowel sounds with no stress on the consonant sounds, but do not articulate sounds artificially in any way.

(6) **Do your best not to repeat sounds, words or anything.** Say what you have to say without repeating at all—and it *is* possible—no matter how you feel about it. Always keep moving forward. If you stutter, stutter forward.[1] When you make a sound there is no use making it over again.[2]—you can and should proceed to the next sound or word.

(7) **Pay attention to the fluent speech you have.** Don't just be aware of your stuttering. Listen to yourself when you are fluent.[3] You need to recognize and remember your successful and pleasant speaking experiences. Feel your fluency.

---

[1]Why continue to make a sound when you have already produced it? (VanRiper)

[2]The stutterer needs to stutter forward. He needs to go ahead . . . without regard to anticipated difficulty. (Sheehan)

[3]Pay more attention to your normal speech than to what you think of as your stuttering. (Johnson)

(8) While working on this program **try to talk as much as you can** since you will need every opportunity to work on the procedures recommended. Talk more— you've been silent long enough. Speak out when you want to.[1,2] If opportunities to talk do not exist you should do your best to make some.

(9) **Try to resist time pressure.**[3] At the moment you are expected to speak, you may have an almost panicky feeling of haste and urgency. You feel that you are under "time pressure" with no time to lose, and you have a compulsive feeling that you must speak quickly without taking the time for deliberate and relaxed expression. Do your best to resist this time pressure feeling.[4] Pause— take your time—there is no hurry. Unless there is a fire —people will wait to hear what you have to say. Make them wait—and don't hurry saying 'hello' on the phone. Pause! Take your time.

These then are the nine ground rules that should govern your behavior as you get ready to do the job that must be done. But how do you achieve these goals? It's easy to be told what to do but it's hard to do it. It's difficult to change the habits and practices of many years. All we say is that it is necessary and the choice is yours.

---

[1]Findings suggest that the more a stutterer talks the better, and the more people he talks to and the more situations he talks in, the better. (Johnson)

[2]The stutterer should be encouraged to talk as much as possible. (Brown)

[3]A basic feature of stuttering behavior is that the stutterer is under time pressure to a great extent. (Sheehan)

[4]Panic, tension, and an overwhelming urgency are the hallmarks of stuttering: they are what you must overcome. Totally resist any feelings of hurry and pressure. Let'em wait. (J. D. Williams)

It is suggested that you check yourself carefully and write down your achievements in your notebook so you can keep a record of how well you control your speech in line with these recommendations.

You might start by using the system of tackling one ground rule at a time, beginning with the first one—speaking slowly and deliberately. First, collect one successful performance, then two in a row, then three in a series, and so on, until you have been able to collect ten consecutive listeners to whom you have spoken slowly and deliberately.

Then similarly, begin to work on the second ground rule—which is most important—in the same way. You should record in your notebook what you have been able to accomplish each day. It would also be helpful if you could tape record at least some of your performance so you can be sure that you are doing it right.

Another way would be to set up a daily quota. The first day collect at least one instance in which you fulfilled the requirements of one ground rule; the next day you try for two and so on. Or you could set up a maximum and minimum quota when you get up in the morning. Then do your collecting as you go about your daily work and make note of your accomplishments in the notebook.

In defining your goals set up a minimum you are sure you can do and a maximum that may strain your motivation and yet be achieved. For example, devise the following for ground rules Nos. 4 and 5—speaking in a strong firm voice with inflection. For a minimum goal "I will use a strong resonant speech while reading aloud to myself for ten minutes"; for maximum goal "I will use it in five phone calls whether I stutter or not". Each day record your performance honestly, and try to cover all of the nine rules. And with each subsequent day gradually increase your quota.

It will not be easy. We know it can be a struggle to follow these guidelines. If you try and fail on some of them, do not get disheartened. Other stutterers have met difficulties and conquered them. Don't give up. If you can only reduce the tension and severity of your struggle behavior by learning to stutter easily and openly (ground rule No. 2) you will have made a lot of progress toward your goal.

After you have done your level best to conform and live up to the ground rules, let's now discuss the subject of finding out what you do when you stutter.

If the stutterer in this book is sometimes referred to as "he" or "him", this may be considered as fairly representative since it is estimated that there are about four times as many male stutterers as there are female.[1]

---

[1]There is less stuttering among girls than among boys. This may be attributed to the fact that girls are better organized than boys . . . this does not mean that females are better organized than males at all periods of life; in fact, females encounter more disorganizing illness than the males at middle age. Yet girls are better organized than boys in the formative period of life. They are more fluent in speech. (Bluemel)

Licking the problem of stuttering, mastering your own mouth, takes time; it cannot be accomplished overnight. How long it will take you I cannot say, for no two stutterers approach the challenge in the same way or move at the same rate but all have in common a beckoning mirage luring them ahead. (Emerick)

Finding Out What You Do
When You Stutter

A fundamental part of this program involves your finding out what you do when you stutter. Therefore we must emphasize how important it is for you to not only identify what you are doing at the moment of stuttering, but also what you do in trying to stop or avoid trouble.[1,2,3] It is essential for you to know what these things are, so you can work at changing or correcting them. And of course you should be particularly concerned about what you do which is unnecessary or abnormal.[4]

In other words we ask that you become sincerely interested in identifying the various kinds of behavior that constitute your stuttering act, particularly those features which can be changed or corrected. Maybe you hate to even think about your stuttering but this information is essential. Your assignments will include first studying the actions you make which may not be directly involved in the formation of speech sounds or words, and then later the specific activity of your speech mechanism when you talk.

To do this you will be asked to stutter on purpose imitating your usual pattern and observe yourself in the

---

[1]Perhaps the first concrete step you should take is to acquaint yourself with your stuttering behavior. (Murray)

[2]Try to identify what you are doing wrong when you stutter. (Emerick)

[3]The stutterer must come to know just what he does when he approaches a feared word or situation. (VanRiper)

[4]When a problem exists, the first thing to do is to examine it carefully with the hope of discovering what is wrong. (Rainey)

mirror[1] while doing it, and make recordings of conversations when you are having trouble. Such assignments may seem weird or abhorrent but you need to face up to and confront your problem no matter how distressing it may be.[2] Others see and hear you stutter and you should be able to stand it if they can. It isn't all that bad anyway.

There would be no way for you to figure out how to control your stuttering if you couldn't identify the specific actions which constitute your stuttering and which can be changed.[3] Besides the more you study and analyze your stuttering the less sensitive you will be about it.

You can then learn to change your abnormal speech behavior by putting into effect controls which will correct or modify what you do wrong. This does not mean that you are going to be told or expected to learn how to talk by consciously manipulating your speech mechanism as that would be impossible but you can at least try to change what you do wrong.

In carrying out this program keep in mind that stuttering is something you are doing; it is not something that happens to you, nor is it some outside mysterious

---

[1]Watching yourself stutter in a mirror makes you more objective and less emotional about your stuttering. (Trotter)

[2]You will have to make yourself do these things and they will not be easy. (LaPorte)

[3]It is important that you learn as much as possible about how you stutter and what you do when you stutter so that you can modify the symptoms. (Boland)

force that manipulates you rendering you helpless.[1] And you can change the way you stutter.

Unfortunately the chances are that you have only a vague idea of how you stutter and probably are unable to correctly duplicate your abnormalities.[2] Possibly all you know is that sometimes you speak freely and at other times you get miserably stuck. We want you to be able to answer the question—what am I doing wrong when I stutter.[3] Of course this will include what your speech muscles do, referring to the muscles you use to control your breath, your mouth, your lips, tongue, etc.[4]

After you have found out what you do when you stutter, then you can compare your behavior at that time with how you act when you speak fluently. From this comparison you will learn what wrong things you do which you can stop and need to eliminate because they are unnecessary.[5]

This information will also give you the opportunity of studying ways and means of changing or correcting

---

[1]It is very good for you to understand clearly that the things you do that interfere with the normally easy flow of your speech are indeed things you do yourself. They do not just happen to you. (Johnson)

[2]Early in my therapy program, I made a startling discovery. Although I had stuttered for years, I really did not know much about what I did with my speech apparatus as I stuttered. (Luper)

[3]You've got to examine and analyze the act of speaking to see what errors you're making. What are you doing wrong that makes your speech come out as stuttering? (Starbuck)

[4]How you stutter is terribly important. (Sheehan)

[5]You will need to eliminate the abnormality of your stuttering and try to find an easier way to talk which is under your control. (Neely)

other things you do incorrectly. And the more you study the errors you make when stuttering, the more confidence you will have that you can lick them.[1] Part of your fear of stuttering is due to its mysteriousness. By observing and studying it objectively some of the fear will decline.

Meanwhile you are asked in the next chapter to be willing to admit that you are a stutterer. And as you start on this step, please remember that you should make a real attempt to accomplish the goal of each step before proceeding to the next one.

---

[1]The better your understanding of your speech problem and of what you yourself are doing that complicates the problem, the more you can do to help yourself feel capable of dealing with it successfully. (Johnson)

Yes, I am a stutterer, and I hope that it will help any stutterer who may read this to know that I was such a severe stutterer that I could not put two meaningful words together until I was twenty-four years old. Do I still stutter? Oh, I call myself a stutterer because I still have small interruptions in my speech now and then. But, there's another more important reason why I call myself a stutterer. I'm not trying to hide the fact anymore! (Rainey)

Admitting That You Stutter

If you are like most stutterers you are constantly afraid that people will find out that you are a stutterer. The amount of energy you may spend in hiding your disorder can be tremendous. Possibly you devise intricate strategies of avoidance and disguise. Or you may assume some kind of a masquerade in the hope, usually a vain one, that your listener won't recognize that you are a stutterer. This burden is a heavy one and it only makes communication more difficult.[1]

Where does all that anxiety and worry get you? Nowhere. It only makes matters worse since it just builds up more fear and tension. And you know that the frequency and severity of your stuttering is in proportion to the amount of fear and tension you have. So what can or should be done about it? Even if you are not obsessed with hiding the fact that you stutter you need to get rid of what worry you have on this point.

The answer is simple but not easy. You can counteract most of that worry and concern by just admitting that you are a stutterer.[2] So this step calls for you to admit to others frankly and willingly that you are a stutterer and stop pretending that you are a normal speaker.

This will take a lot of courage on your part, but this needs to be done as it is important for you to reduce your sensitivity about your stuttering. It will pay off to do so. It's no disgrace to be a stutterer anyway. You may think so, but you are wrong if you do.

---

[1]No problem is solved by denying its existence. (Brown)

[2]You will remain a stutterer as long as you continue to pretend not to be one. (Sheehan)

You can not afford to allow yourself to be so over-come by hypersensitivity that you are afraid to discuss your problem.[1] If you are afraid to talk about your stuttering and can not confront it openly, it will be hard for you to remain calm enough and retain sufficient self-control to work according to our recommendations. Don't allow your feelings to defeat your efforts. Resist the urge to hide your stuttering.

This request does not mean that you should blurt out immediately to everyone that you are a stutterer or make unnecessary announcements of this fact even though that attitude might be helpful. Still you should not shirk this assignment. You should make occasion to freely admit to those with whom you associate and with whom you normally talk that you are a stutterer and be willing to discuss it with them.

Start on this assignment by talking with people you are close to. Then increase the number of people you can discuss it with until you find that you have no hesitancy in talking about stuttering with anyone.[2, 3]

For example, you could say to a friend something to the effect that "you know that I am a stutterer and frankly I have been ashamed to admit it and I need to be more open and frank about my problem and may need your help." Any real friend will appreciate your frank-

---

[1]If you are like all of the other adult stutterers I have known, you create, without meaning to, of course—a major share of any adjustment difficulties you may have . . . by trying to cover up, conceal or disguise the fact that you talk the way you do. (Johnson)

[2]Whenever you have an opportunity to discuss your stuttering with someone, do it! (LaPorte)

[3]You need to communicate more openly and easily with other people including being frank about your stuttering. (Boland)

ness and will feel closer to you as a result. Besides you will find that people are interested in stuttering. Teach them about it.

This is not an easy assignment but complying with it will reduce your tension. And it will help you accept your stuttering as a problem with which you can cope with less shame and embarrassment. This can make a world of difference in enabling you to adopt that more healthy, wholesome and objective attitude toward your difficulty which all stutterers need so badly.

If you frankly admit you are a stutterer you may think it will hurt your pride, but it is more likely that you will be proud of yourself for doing it. Besides there is no use spending your life pretending.[1, 2]

Of course you can't accomplish this goal in a day or two. It will take time to make contact with people you know and carry out this recommendation. No matter how long it takes, it will help reduce your tension and fear if you cultivate the attitude of being willing to talk about your stuttering.

Can you do so? As the fellow said "it ain't easy"— and that's putting it mildly. It may be far from easy— in fact it can be tough.

This is a very beneficial step toward relieving you of

---

[1] Murder will out, and so will stuttering. (VanRiper)

[2] Your fear of stuttering is based largely on your shame and hatred of it. The fear is also based on playing the phony role of pretending your stuttering doesn't exist. (Sheehan)

much of your fear and tension and is most necessary. If you are determined you can do it. If you can't make up your mind to tackle this assignment, it may not be worth the trouble to read any further unless you are just interested in finding out how this therapy program works.[1]

Voluntary Stuttering

In working on this first step it is suggested that occasionally you should stutter voluntarily. Stutterers can usually get relief from fear and tension by doing this. If you deliberately stutter, you directly attack and help to reduce the tension which is aggravating your problem by voluntarily doing that which you dread.[2]

Voluntary stuttering sometimes called fake or pseudo stuttering, should take the form of easy simple repetitions or short prolongations of the first sound or syllable of a word or the word itself. It should be done only on non-feared words in a calm and relaxed manner. Do not imitate your own pattern of stuttering but stutter in a different way.[3, 4]

Whatever type of easy stuttering you decide to use, you must be sure to keep it entirely voluntary as you

---

[1]A major problem in the treatment of stuttering is how to encourage the stutterer to stay in and continue with the course of treatment. (Barbara)

[2]When the stutterer does voluntary stuttering, he can say to himself "I am doing the thing I fear. Also I realize that I can change my speech; I can tell my speech mechanism what to do." (Gregory)

[3]Deliberately stutter! Yes, stutter on purpose in as many situations as possible, but stutter in a different way. (LaPorte)

[4]Even if he feels beforehand that he can speak without stuttering, the stutterer is encouraged to pretend or fake stuttering—but to do so in a way different from his usual manner of stuttering. (Barbara)

can not afford to let it get out of control and become involuntary. Purposely experiment talking slowly and deliberately with easy repetitions or prolongations that differ from your usual pattern. It will give you a sense of self-mastery when you control the uncontrollable.

You could start when alone by reading aloud and calmly making easy repetitions and prolongations. Then later you can work it into conversations with others. Make up some assignments for yourself in which you are required to stutter voluntarily.[1] For instance, go into a store and ask the clerk the cost of different items, faking blocks on the word "cost". Make the blocks easy but obvious.

Voluntary stuttering will help eliminate your shame and embarrassment. The more you can follow through and practice doing this, the easier it will become. Aim toward the goal of being willing to stutter without becoming emotionally disturbed.[2]

---

[1]One means of satisfying the fear of stuttering is to stutter voluntarily on nonfeared words in all kinds of situations. This has the effect of helping you reduce the pressure that you feel when you try to avoid stuttering, and of enabling you to handle your speech more effectively. (Sheehan)

[2]Now I am going to ask you to do a strange thing: *to stutter on purpose.* I know it sounds weird but it works. Why? Because it helps drain away the fear (what have you got to hide if you are willing to stutter on purpose?) and it provides a lot of experience practicing the act of stuttering in a highly voluntary and purposeful manner. The more you stutter on purpose, the less you hold back; and the less you hold back, the less you stutter. (Emerick)

Work at it for several reasons. It is one way of admitting that you are a stutterer. It is also a way of finding out how people react to stuttering and will help you realize that they are usually kind and tolerant. And it will give you the satisfaction of knowing that you have the courage to tackle your handicap in an obvious way.[1]

It would also be helpful if you could inject a little humor or even be willing to joke about your stuttering.[2] To do this would definitely help reduce your sensitivity. One way, as discussed, would call for you to voluntarily stutter on purpose.

Or, occasionally, you could make some joking remark about your stuttering[3]—such as, explaining that if you didn't talk you wouldn't stutter—or just say, in response to some emphatic explanation "you tell him, I stutter"—or announce "there may be a brief intermission due to technical difficulties". These remarks aren't very funny, are they? Probably, not to you as a stutterer, but they could be to others.

---

[1] By gradually learning to stutter on purpose and without pain, (the stutterer) will lose a lot of the negative emotions that color his disorder; when this occurs, he'll find great relief. (VanRiper)

[2] Consider humor as you look at your mistakes in speaking. Many things about stuttering can be funny. (Neely)

[3] One way to make your listener feel at ease about your stuttering is to tell an occasional joke about it. (Trotter)

It would be just great if you could develop a sense of humor about your difficulty.[1] At the same time do not go overboard and laughingly and fraudulently pretend that your stuttering is funny, as some stutterers have done, while feeling terrible about it inside.

A stutterer's willingness to stutter, particularly in a modified way, is a very powerful psychological aspect of therapy that can lead to a most lasting and satisfying change in fluency.

---

[1]Make fun of your stuttering and yourself. The best of all humor is self-directed. (Emerick)

You might be interested in a quotation by a non-stutterer from a letter written many years ago by Thomas Carlyle, the historian, to Ralph Waldo Emerson, dated November 17, 1843. He said "a stammering man is never a worthless one . . . It is an excess of delicacy, excess of sensibility to the presence of his fellow-creature, that makes his stammer". Even in those days they realized that sensitivity was an important factor in actuating and maintaining stuttering.

Eliminating Secondary Symptoms

This next step affects one factor involved in finding out what you do when you stutter. It calls for you to eliminate—that is, stop doing—the unnecessary or accessory movements which may characterize your particular pattern of stuttering. You may be surprised to find out that you have several of these.

We do not refer to the actions of your speech muscles but to other unnatural mannerisms or habits which you have acquired and have become part of your stuttering behavior. They are what speech pathologists call secondary symptoms and refer to actions which are not necessary in the production of speech.

These include movements such as eye blinks, closings or fixations, facial or mouth grimaces, covering your mouth with your hand, head tossing or scratching, jaw jerks, ear pulling, finger snapping or tapping, coin jingling, knee slapping, foot tapping or shuffling, arm swinging*, hand movements or what have you.[1,2]

Any such unnecessary actions probably started because at one time they helped you get through a block

---

*Normal gesturing is not objectional—in fact is encouraged—provided it is not timed to the beat of the word or syllable for the purpose of avoiding stuttering.

[1]Become aware of head or arm movements, eye blinking, other movements or body rigidity, lip smacking or other noises, puffing of the cheeks or pressing the lips. (Moses)

[2]John's habitual pattern consisted of a violent tilting back of his head; rolling his eyes toward the ceiling; the muscles in his neck would stand out: he would become flushed; he would twist his face in a forced grimace; attempt various starters; some head jerks in an effort to release himself from the blocks and would also accompany his stuttering with various body gestures. (Sheehan)

or enabled you to hide or avoid trouble. But now they may have become part of the stuttering itself. You will be happier to be free of these unnecessary and unattractive actions.

Of course you are not guilty of doing all these things but you should get rid of any habits of this type you may have. You need to learn how to control them.[1,2] But before you can tackle them, it is necessary to know what they are which, of course, involves finding out what you do when you stutter.

It is difficult to scrutinize yourself and be fully aware of habits which you have been using to avoid difficulty and which you have accumulated over the years. Normally you cannot see yourself stuttering but you should be able to feel what you do. Possibly you can imitate your stuttering in front of a mirror. Or ask a member of your family or a close friend to watch when you stutter and make notes after you have described what to look for.

You could start by picking out in advance some specific speaking situations which will occur today or tomorrow. Resolve to study yourself as carefully as possible on these occasions, looking out for unnecessary movements you make when stuttering or when expecting to. Disregard any normal gestures, making sure they are normal and not used to beat time with the speech at-

---

[1]He (the stutterer) will learn, much to his surprise that these secondary symptoms are not an integral part of his disorder, that it is possible for him to stutter without using them. (VanRiper)

[2]When these reactions are recognized as secondary symptoms, they can gradually be minimized and controlled and the stammerer is then in a better position to contend with the primary speech disorder. (Bluemel)

tempt or to jerk out of your stutter. After each situation make a list of the symptoms in your notebook.[1]

Probably you will have little trouble identifying and listing the more conspicious ones but it may be more difficult to spot others. Very often stutterers are quite unaware of behaviors that may be obvious to others. Watch yourself carefully on several occasions. You may be surprised to find you are doing things that you would not do if you weren't expecting to stutter.

Here's where a mirror, particularly a full-length mirror will come in handy to help you observe yourself. Assuming you have difficulty talking on the telephone, make some phone calls while watching yourself in the mirror.[2] Make notes of any or all irregular movements (or postures) associated with your stuttering. Don't skip any of them. What did you find? To double check, make a phone call which will be embarrassing and will put pressure on you. Did you note anything different on this call?

Now comes the hard part, how do you go about eliminating these behaviors? Sometimes such habits can be so compulsive that they are seemingly almost impossible to stop. But you can stop them, if you make up your mind to do so. You can't stop stuttering by willpower, but if you are determined you can get rid of secondary

---

[1]Begin by listing the struggle behavior that you use and which are not part of the act of speaking. Recognize and specify what you do when you stutter. Begin by listing the struggle behaviors that you use which are not part of the act of speaking. You will seek to eliminate these behaviors by increasing your awareness of them and separating them from your attempts to talk. (Moses)

[2]For example, you can look at yourself in the mirror and assess what you are doing while you make a phone call likely to elicit stuttering. (Murray)

symptoms by disciplining yourself to do so. But you will need to go about it in a systematic manner.

Suggested Assignments—How to Go About It

See page 113 where a systematic procedure is outlined, describing how to go about eliminating secondary symptoms. Getting rid of all your secondary symptoms must be your definite goal.[1] It can be done. In doing this you will be getting rid of crutches which may have originally helped you get the word out but which can give no permanent relief.[2] And you should not proceed to the next step until you feel that you have mastered this part of your problem.

Enlisting the Support of Others

In the foregoing discussion it was suggested that you might have a member of your family or a close friend help you become aware of any secondary symptoms you have. Someone like that, acting as an observer should be able to see or hear things you may not be aware of, but this person should know what to look for.

At the same time we would emphasize that this is a program of self-therapy and it has been planned on the assumption that you may not have anyone to whom you can turn for specialized help. Therefore the success of

---

[1] Get rid of these artificial devices! This may seem impossible at first, but depend on your own natural resources and you will find that in the final analysis you will be greatly rewarded. (Barbara)

[2] The job is to think and work in a positive manner. The job involves coming to realize that these head jerks, eye blinks, tongue clicks . . . are not helping to get those words out. They are preventing the words from being said strongly, aggressively and fluently. (Rainey)

this program can not be dependent on anyone but yourself.[1]

However, this does not mean that you should refuse assistance. If you have a relative or friend with whom you have a good and trusting relationship, someone you have confidence in, he or she can render you valuable service in many ways.[2]

Such a person might help you monitor your speech, accompany you on some of your assignments, compliment you on your efforts, give you moral support and encourage you to carry on and persevere until you reach your goal. You need all the encouragement you can get.[3]

(Sometimes friends with the best of intentions offer unsolicited advice about what they have heard or think you should do to overcome your stuttering. Although such advice may be unwanted, it is suggested that it should be accepted gracefully even though it is based on an inadequate understanding of what is causing the difficulty.)

---

[1]The stutterer must get out of his mind that he can be "cured" by somebody else. (Wedberg)

[2]What I needed was not an authority but a friend and collaborator genuinely interested in me and ready to help me. I was fortunate to have a brother who could be this friend. (Freund)

[3]My high school chemistry teacher, a former stutterer, gave up his lunch hour twice a week to talk with me about speech . . . Perhaps you can find this kind of sympathetic friend who will listen while you talk about your stuttering. Let him know that you do not expect advice. You don't expect him to be clinician, just a friend. (Brown)

Avoidance is the heart and core of stuttering. Avoidance behavior—holding back—is essential for the maintainance of stuttering behavior. Stuttering simply cannot survive a total weakening of avoidance, coupled with a concerted strengthening of approach tendencies. If there is no holding back there is no stuttering. What distinguishes all stuttering behavior? A holding back. And what happens in situations in which the stutterer doesn't care? He becomes fluent. (Sheehan)

Eliminating
Avoidances and Postponements

Now that you willingly admit that you are a stutterer and have done your best to eliminate your secondary symptoms you are ready for the next step. This *most important* next step calls for you to make a real effort to eliminate—that means stop—any and all avoidance or postponement habits or tricks which you may have acquired to put off, hide or minimize your stuttering.

This may present more of a problem than you think, since much of a stutterer's abnormal behavior may be traced to his efforts to postpone or avoid what he considers threatening situations.[1] Probably you think that you must be ready for every eventuality so you can either avoid the danger of stuttering entirely or meet it fully prepared. You may feel that being caught unprepared is the worst thing that can happen to you so you do your best to postpone and avoid anticipated trouble.[2,3]

While temporarily affording relief, avoidance or postponement tactics actually increase your fear and cause you more trouble in the long run. For instance, if the

---

[1]The stutterer believes that the most important part of communication in speech is to avoid stuttering at all costs. (Trotter)

[2]Working on my own I set about to eliminate every last vestige of avoidance of words and situations. (Sheehan)

[3]Like many of you, one of the most common and debilitating characteristics of my problem was the habit of avoiding . . . There was almost no limit to what I would do to avoid situations in which I feared my stuttering would embarrass me. Going to a party would be an extremely tiring event because the entire evening would be spent trying to stay alert for words on which I might stutter and finding ways to avoid them. (Luper)

telephone rings and you refuse to answer, because you are afraid you won't be able to talk well, the act of avoiding this situation will only tend to build up your fear of the telephone.[1] Avoidances have been described as a pump in the reservoir of fear. They keep it aroused until time runs out or their effectiveness wears out. You need to quit running and hiding.[2, 3, 4] Postponements are bad enough but avoidances are worse though they are often interchangeable.

Postponements include stalling devices such as clearing your throat, swallowing, coughing, blowing your nose, putting in unnecessary words such as 'you know' or 'I mean' or 'that is' or making excessive use of interjections like 'uh', 'er', 'well', and so on. This includes repeating preceding words, prolonging the tail end of the preceding word and slowing down the rate at which the preceding words are spoken. It is particularly unwise to postpone occasions when you should talk—more on that later.

---

[1]I remember well how often I "played-deaf" when the telephone would ring. Sometimes, unfortunately, I might be standing not more than a few feet from the ringing telephone and my protestations regarding "answer that telephone" would be of no avail. (Adler)

[2]We never conquer fear by running away from it; we only increase it. (VanRiper)

[3]Avoidance can be defined as a process of shying away from the responsibility of facing your problems. (La Porte)

[4]You must sharply reduce or eliminate the avoidances you use. Everytime you substitute one word for another, use a sound or some trick to get speech started, postpone or give up an attempt at talking, you make it harder for yourself. (Emerick)

Substituting synonyms, easy words or phrases for the ones on which you think you will block is now taboo.[1, 2, 3] Nor should you try to sneak up on a feared word from a different direction or adopt other strategies of substitution. Similarly, you should not try to avoid trouble by varying the pitch, or intensity of your voice, by speaking more rapidly or repeating, by going back and getting a running start, by talking in a monotone or sing-song way, by any sort of unnatural speech, such as whispered rehearsal, or by acting like a clown or affecting unnaturally aggressive behavior.

As you identify the avoidance or postponement tricks you have been using list them in your notebook as you did for your secondary symptoms. The list will help you watch out for and stop using them.

Please be honest with yourself about your avoidances.[4] You should not pretend you don't hear when

---

[1]In shunning difficult words the stammerer has recourse to synonyms, circumlocutions and evasions. With the adult stutterer the use of synonyms becomes a standard method of escaping the speech impediment . . . One stammerer says facetiously that he has learned the whole dictionary in order to have synonyms available. (Bluemel)

[2]At times you may totally avoid stuttering by choosing to be absent, by withdrawing from a speaking situation, or while speaking you may substitute a non-feared word (one on which you do not expect to stutter) for a feared one. This allows you to escape for the moment, but increases the worry about future situations. (J. D. Williams)

[3]The thing that discouraged me most was the realization that I could no longer detour around a difficult bugaboo word with the substitution of a clever synonym. (Wedberg)

[4]The stutterer should develop a conscience which itself will penalize the tendency to avoid. (VanRiper)

someone speaks to you.[1] You should not stand mute pretending to think of the answer, nor say you do not know when you do know. You should not dodge speaking situations or avoid social responsibilities or give up speech attempts or leave the scene of approaching trouble.[2]

Possibly you may even have turned down a job opportunity or career because you thought it would call for too much talking. It's not necessary to run away. Actually, wouldn't you derive a sense of achievement by voluntarily entering feared situations which would help you foster a sense of pride in your ability to get along without avoidances?

This does not mean that you need to volunteer to make speeches before an audience, but you will feel better if you don't avoid normal opportunities to speak out. You need to talk as much as possible.[3] As you progress you will be encouraged to enter many situations that offer a challenge. Sooner or later you will have to stop retreating.[4] The sooner the better.

As has been pointed out, stuttering is largely what the stutterer does trying not to stutter (avoidance).[5] So

---

[1]You sometimes create the impression of aloofness, or unfriendliness, or stupidity when you are in reality, friendly and well-informed. (Johnson)

[2]Don't avoid certain words or situations that trigger stuttering. Face them head-on. It's far better to stutter than to avoid speaking situations because the fear of stuttering just compounds the problem. (Murray)

[3]Enter more speaking situations. (D. Williams)

[4]Avoidance only increases fear and stuttering and must be reduced. (Czuchna)

[5]Your pattern of stuttering behavior consists chiefly of the things you are doing to avoid stuttering. (J. D. Williams)

if you could wholeheartedly adopt an attitude of not wanting to avoid, it would make a world of difference in the amount of trouble you have.[1]

Suggested Assignments—How To Go About It

This vital step requires concentrated effort as it sure is not easy as you need help. It is suggested that you read, study and put to work assignments such as those listed on page 117. Turn to that page.

When you have gotten rid of your secondary symptoms and stopped your avoidance and postponement tricks you will have eliminated most of the by-products and unnecessary features which your fears have engendered. Please be sure you have done your best on this assignment before starting on the next step.

---

[1]Determine to reduce your use of avoidances. (Moses)

If a stutterer is going to change radically his accustomed manner of stuttering, he must work persistently and diligently over a long period of time. (Johnson)

Maintaining Eye Contact

If you are like many stutterers you do not look people squarely in the eye when you talk to them. Chances are that if you observe yourself carefully you will find that you usually avert your eyes particularly when you are stuttering or anticipating a block. And by doing so you only increase any shame you might already feel and furthermore you lose touch with your audience.

So this step in therapy calls for you to establish the habit of eye contact with those you talk to. This doesn't mean that you should stare fixedly at the person to whom you are talking, but still you should look the other person squarely in the eye more or less continuously. Establish eye contact before you begin to speak and continue to do so in a natural way.[1] Particularly do your best not to look away when you stutter or expect to.

It is possible that you already practice good eye contact but more probably you are so shy that you do not. Remember that it is difficult for you to observe yourself, so do your best to be sincerely honest with yourself. Possibly you should ask someone with whom you converse, such as a member of your family, to watch to find out if you shift your eyes just before or when you stutter.

Perhaps you look away because you are afraid that your listener will react with pity, rejection or impatience, which is not apt to be true. By using eye contact it will enable you to test the validity of your fears and it should put your listener more at ease. Moreover by maintaining eye contact you can demonstrate that you are accepting —not rejecting—your stuttering, as a problem to be

---

[1]You must acquire the ability to keep good eye contact with your listener throughout your moment of stuttering. (VanRiper)

71

solved.[1] When you look away you are denying the problem.

Anyway, you should do your best to maintain good eye contact as a habit.[2] You will feel better for doing so, as it will help you combat feelings of inadequacy and embarrassment. Psychiatrists recommend it in trying to help people who are shy and bashful. Interpersonal communication is facilitated by eye contact even if you didn't stutter.[3] Good speakers use it naturally.

It is unnecessary for you to turn or hang your head in shame which may be what you are doing unconsciously when you avert your eyes. You should try to develop a feeling of confidence that you are as good as the next person and do your best to look the world squarely in the eye.

Suggested Assignments

It's easier said than done. See recommendations on page 123 as to how you can go about training yourself to maintain eye contact.

---

[1]The value of eye contact is the effect it has on the stutterer. It almost forces him to keep the stuttering going forward through the word. It's an assertive behavior and a positive act. It's hard to withdraw and back off if you are holding eye contact. (Starbuck)

[2]Establish eye contact before you begin to speak. Two or three seconds of quiet eye contact can get you off to a better start. (Sheehan)

[3]Try to maintain eye contact with your listeners. Looking away severs the communication link with your audience and convinces them that you are ashamed and disgusted with the way you talk. (Moses)

What Comes Next

Of course there is no way for us to know what progress you have been able to make in this program. However it would be most commendable if it could be assumed that you have changed your speaking behavior by letting your speech be continually governed according to the recommendations set by the ground rules.

To the extent that this has been done it should have made a substantial difference. Even if you only complied with one of the rules—such as talking easily and openly —you should be able to communicate with less stress and strain.

Then if it could also be assumed that you followed through on the recommendations described in the last four chapters, it would mean that you now willingly admit that you are a stutterer; that your secondary symptoms have been eliminated; that you maintain good eye contact; and that you have discontinued all your old avoidance habits and practices.

Possibly it would be too much to expect completely satisfactory observance or compliance with all these objectives, but surely you should now be able to look at your problem less emotionally and more objectively, and should have cleared away any entangling obstacles which may have complicated your disorder.

What comes next? Hopefully you are now an "honest" stutterer, stuttering without any useless accessory frills, etc.[1] So the next step will call for you to investigate

---

[1]The first thing you must become is an honest stutterer. (Starbuck)

what your speech mechanism is doing abnormally at the instant you block.

After you have studied and analyzed what your speech muscles are doing improperly at that time you are asked to put into effect post-block and pre-block corrections. These corrections are designed to enable you to move smoothly in a predetermined manner through those sounds and words which may give you trouble. This will complete the program.

Therapy must be practiced full time to be highly successful. You must feel that you are on the right track and you must be committed to putting the program into practice. Plan your work well, then work your plan harder than you have ever worked before. Success will follow. (Boehmler)

Analyzing Your Blocks

In this step you are asked to explore what you do wrong with your speech mechanism when you are stuttering.[1] Continue to keep in mind that stuttering is something you are doing[2] and that you can change what you are doing. We want you to be able to answer the question—what am I doing with my speech muscles when I stutter?

This refers to the muscles you use to control your breath, your mouth, your lips, tongue, etc. You need to become familiar with the abnormal speech muscle movements which take place when you block.[3] The more you study your stuttering behavior the more you will realize that you can change it.[4]

---

[1]Look and listen closely and discover just what it is that you are doing when you stutter. (Rainey)

[2]Stuttering is a series of activities you do. (Emerick)

[3]At a time when you feel that you "are stuttering" pay very close attention to what you are doing . . . You can ask yourself—precisely what are you doing? You should answer this question in descriptive detail, and when you have done this you should always ask yourself why you were doing what you were doing. (Johnson)

[4]All of us know that this process of confronting yourself will not be pleasant but we also know you will find, as you observe and analyze what you do and feel when stuttering or expecting to stutter, that you will then know what you have to change. (VanRiper)

To Make a Comparison

After you discover what you are letting your speech muscles do abnormally when you stutter, you will be able to compare their activity then with the way they act when you speak fluently.[1] From this comparison you can figure out ways and means of correcting or changing your faulty speech muscle behavior.[2, 3]

Making this comparison between your good and bad speech would be easy if you knew exactly how to imitate the way you stutter. But, unfortunately as has been previously discussed, it is most unlikely that you can do this, because practically all stutterers can not do so unless or until they have carefully studied their own stuttering pattern.[4, 5]

---

[1]You, as a stutterer, must study your speech patterns in order to become aware of the differences between stuttered and fluent speech. (Neely)

[2]Once you begin to see what you are doing that makes talking difficult, you will find that much of this behavior is controllable. (Luper)

[3]It is helpful for the stutterer to learn to analyze and identify the specific movements or lack of movements involved in his stuttering behavior. He will learn this by attending carefully to his behavior, e.g. what he is doing with his tongue, jaw and lips as he is stuttering. Then he can have a basis for comparison between what he needs to do to talk and what he is doing to interfere with that process. Most importantly, he can learn that he is doing things to interfere with talking, and hence he can learn to change them. (D. Williams)

[4]Odd as this may seem, few severe stutterers know what they are doing that interferes with the forward flow of speech. (Johnson)

[5]To ask a stutterer to begin immediately to change the way he stutters is to ask for failure, if only because he rarely knows how he stutters. (VanRiper)

As a result you need to conduct a self-examination and try to monitor your blocks so you can develop a feeling or sense of awareness of the movement and positions of your speech mechanism during stuttering.[1]

(Obviously for this purpose you need to continue to stutter, so don't stop now! You need every opportunity to get the feedback from your speech behavior.)

All right, how do you conduct this self-examination? One way to get that feeling of what is happening is for you to stutter extremely slowly when you block. This does not mean that you have to talk slowly—just stutter that way. When you anticipate trouble, go ahead and stutter but do it in such slow motion that you have time to feel exactly what your speech muscles are doing.[2]

Keep on doing this as you consciously try to sense what is happening as you block and in making the transition to the next sound until you are fully aware of what you are doing on those sounds which give you trouble. Make notes of the things you do that are unusual and not necessary.[3] Keep this information for later use.

---

[1]Perhaps the first concrete step you should take is to acquaint yourself with your stuttering behavior . . . In order to carry this out effectively, you must first learn to keep in touch with yourself during your moments of stuttering . . . Feedback of various types will assist you in this self-study endeavor. (Murray)

[2]A simple way to apply this principle in the treatment of stuttering is to have the stutterer maintain or prolong or continue any given position of the speech mechanism that may occur at any stage of what he terms stuttering. (Johnson)

[3]As honestly as you can, try to observe yourself and write down your observations. (J. D. Williams)

Another way to get this information would be to repeat your blocks when you have trouble. If you can screw up your courage, stutter on them over again. But the second time, go through the block in slow motion so that you feel precisely how your speech muscles characteristically behave when you are having trouble.

Using Tape Recorder and Mirror[1]

Your tape recorder can be of real service in studying the way you stutter so that you can imitate it correctly. After you have become familiar with its operation, start recording conversations in situations where you might stutter.[2] This unit should be small and inconspicuous and its use should not be embarrassing—in fact the average person would be interested in observing how it works.

You might begin by making a recording while talking to members of your family. If you have a close friend ask him to let you record while talking with him. Later take the recorder out with you and record as you talk with those with whom you may have difficulty. You will

---

[1]In short, you need to develop a sharp sense of contrast between what you are doing that you call stuttering and what you do as you just talk easily. Use a mirror or a tape recorder to help you observe what you are doing. (D. Williams)

[2]It is possible to record your speech in a communicative stressful situation, then play the tape back for the purpose of careful analysis. Painful as this may seem, it is a good way to bring yourself to grips with your problem. (Murray)

need many recordings of your blocks so you can play them back and listen to yourself.[1, 2]

If you do not want to talk to people you know, then make opportunities to start conversations with strangers even if only to ask the time of day or directions as you make recordings.[3] After you record conversations during the day, then listen to them that night studying and analyzing what you did when you stuttered.

If it is difficult for you to get satisfactory recordings outside the home and you have trouble talking on the phone, move your mirror close to the telephone and start recording phone conversations.[4] Even if you do not have a recorder, talking on the phone in front of a mirror will help you see and feel how you block,[5] provided of course that you stutter in slow motion while talking. As you watch and encounter a block, you might freeze your articulation or continue the repetition, if that is what

---

[1] Listen to recordings of your speech. (Agnello)

[2] I would recommend the almost constant use of a tape recorder. There's nothing like being able to hear your own speech in order to judge what you do and don't like about it, and to decide what changes to make as you practice. Try to record your speech in different situations. (J. D. Williams)

[3] Another classic situation most stutterers fear is asking questions of strangers . . . What I did, and have my patients do, is to stop people who are walking somewhere, or are in stores, and ask them questions concerning the time, directions, the price of some object, etc. (Adler)

[4] For example you can look at yourself in a mirror and assess what you are doing while you make a phone call likely to elicit stuttering. (Murray)

[5] Listen to your own recording of this on tape and watch your performance of it in the mirror . . . By listening to yourself stutter you accustom yourself to the sound of your stuttering. When you are in a real speaking situation and you hear yourself stutter, you're not as likely to panic. (**Trotter**)

you are doing. The idea is to hold your abnormalities long enough to study your actions or postures.

In any case watch yourself in the mirror as you phone stores or offices asking for detailed information while monitoring your stutter.[1] After the call, play back the recording, emphasizing the part where you block. As you repeatedly do this, mimic (silently) or pantomime the actions of your speech muscles along with the recording. You need to see and hear but mainly feel what you are doing as you stutter. Work at this as best you can even if you have no recorder.

Making the Comparison

After you have completed your investigation, you are ready to compare your fluent speech with your stuttered speech. Start by picking out a word that is apt to give you trouble.[2] For instance it might be your name. Anyway, such a word will have a sound in it on which you frequently block.

As you observe yourself in the mirror, stutter purposely on the word imitating the way you get stuck, making the block as realistic as possible.[3] Then repeat the block stuttering on the sound or syllable only, but this time in extremely slow motion. It may be difficult to slow the stuttering down but keep working at it until

---

[1] Use a mirror or a tape recorder to help you observe what you are doing. (D. Williams)

[2] Choose some words that begin with sounds that you think of as being hard—those on which you often stutter. (Aten)

[3] It turns out that a practical way for the stutterer to observe his own stuttering behavior is simply to duplicate it on purpose, imitate it, perform it, while watching himself in the mirror. (Johnson)

you can. Try to get that feeling of awareness of exactly what happens as you block on the sound and in making the transition to the next sound.

Now in order to make the comparison utter the same sound again but correctly, trying to feel what happens when you produce the sound without stuttering as you look in the mirror. Say the syllable in slow motion many times until you become aware of the difference between your speech muscle activity when you block on it and when you say it fluently. Make notes of those things you do that are different, not normal or unnecessary when you stutter.

This may appear complex but it should not be too difficult since you will probably find out that the way you stutter doesn't vary very much You may find that your pattern of stuttering is more or less uniform and consistent since most stutterers tend to repeat the same abnormal postures or speech muscle movements each time they stutter.

Completing this step will take a substantial amount of time but keep at it until you feel you understand what you do incorrectly when you stutter.

Results from Comparison

Now that you have studied your speech behavior in detail and have found out the difference between your good and bad speech, what can you do about it? Part of the answer should now be rather obvious.

From the comparison you have probably discovered that you are making some senseless or unnecessary speech muscle movements and that these are causing part of your difficulty. These movements have nothing to do with the production of the sounds or words you are trying to utter. So you can now work on eliminating any such superfluous or needless actions since you know what they are.

Then try to figure out what you can do to change or modify other abnormal actions you make when uttering the various sounds on which you block. You now know what these are too and can work on changing them.[1] Unfortunately we can not tell you exactly what needs to be done in your case because we are not familiar with the way you stutter. Besides there are so many variations that it would be impossible to describe all of them.

You can not consciously control all the actions involved, but you can try to change or modify those incorrect habits you have built into your speech. If you do this, it will at least make it obvious that you do not need to stutter as you have been doing in the past.

Suggested Assignments—How To Go About It

In the supplement to this chapter we supply information describing not only how you study your speech muscle behavior but also how you work on changing it. To complete this assignment please read and be guided by the assignments listed on page 125, entitled How To Work On Analyzing Your Blocks.

Working to acquire the desired information of this step will take careful analysis but the more insight you have about your difficulty the easier it will be to solve it. In the next step we will explain how to put this information to work. We remind you again that your stuttering is something you are doing and you can change what you are doing.

---

[1]When a moment of stuttering occurs it can be studied and its evil effects erased as much as possible. (Czuchna)

Post-Block Correction

In the last step you studied your stuttering and compared it with your fluent speech. As a result of this study you discovered some, if not all of the errors you make with your speech mechanism that activate or aggravate your blocking.[1] From these observations you should now realize what you do that is abnormal. Hopefully too, you have been able to figure out what you can do to eliminate or at least change some of these abnormalities.

In this step you are to put into effect the results of this study by practicing what are called post-block corrections, sometimes referred to as cancellations.[2] These are pre-determined modifications of the way you stutter, designed to enable you to practice better and more fluent ways of moving through words on which you have had trouble.

After you stutter on a word you are to pause and rehearse corrections that will help you move through a block without difficulty. And a good time to apply these controls is just after you have had a moment of stuttering since there is usually some let-down in tension at that time.

We realize that when you are talking to people it will be embarrassing for you to have to pause and make corrections. Nevertheless that is what you will be asked to do because that is the most effective method of prac-

---

[1]Stutterers need to learn what to do when they do stutter if they are to eventually reduce the fear and frustration involved. (Czuchna)

[2]You must learn how to cancel. This refers to a technique wherein you go right through your old stuttering block, then pause during which you study the block you have just had, then try the word in a different way. (VanRiper)

ticing post-block corrections. Please do your best to follow through on this even though compliance may not be possible every time you stutter. But it is essential that in working this assignment you should put as much effort into it as you can. And you will find that it will not be as embarrassing as you might think.

Briefly it works as follows. After you have stuttered on a word, you first pause and try to calm yourself—then you analyze the block you just had, shifting into slow motion and repeat the whole word in a slow sliding prolonged manner. The extreme slowness is to give you time to make the corrections you need to make while saying it. Your slow speech is to be confined to the word on which you blocked although there may be some carry-over. You are not to talk in that way generally.

In making post-block corrections you are to exaggerate or overcorrect your faulty speech muscle movements. (For example if you block in making the T sound with your tongue stuck to the roof of your mouth, almost reverse your action by hardly letting your tongue touch the roof of your mouth at all.) These or similar corrections are discussed in detail in the chapter on analyzing your blocks and particularly in its supplement.

The following section outlines the sequence of action. Read and study the explanation carefully to be sure that you understand exactly how the process is executed. And then put it into effect when you stutter. Please follow directions—the numbers in parentheses denote the steps in sequence.

Post-Block Correction—Sequence of Action

When you stutter on a word, the first thing you do is (1) finish saying the word on which you have blocked—

i.e., complete the entire word.[1] Don't quit or use a trick to dodge it. Then (2) you have got to have the guts to pause—come to a complete stop, once the word has been uttered. The pause will give you time to study your problem and plan its solution.

Despite time pressure and the feeling that you must keep going, force yourself to rest a moment.[2] Your willingness to stop will help convince yourself as well as your listener that you are determined to be in control of the situation. Furthermore resisting time pressure helps reduce tension.

After you stop, (3) try to relax the tension in your speech mechanism, particularly in your throat. Get the feeling of your tongue lying limp in the bottom of your mouth. Let your jaw drop slightly open as if you were going to drool with your lips loose. The key is to feel the tension draining out as your breathing returns to normal.[3]

As you relax (4) think back and ask yourself what caused you to get stuck on that sound—what did you do wrong—what did you do that was abnormal.[4] In the last step you studied the mistakes you made when you

---

[1]We therefore insist that once the stutterer begins his stutter, he continues until the entire word has been uttered before he cancels it. (VanRiper)

[2]As soon as the stutterer is able to be fairly consistent in pausing after his moment of stuttering, we ask him next to use the pause as an opportunity to try to calm himself and to begin the next word slowly. (VanRiper)

[3]Thinking of and striving for increased relaxation when under stress will provide a competing response which will help you be more calm. (Gregory)

[4]When the word is completed, stop completely and analyze all of the errors you made while all of the tensions and pressures are still fresh. (Starbuck)

blocked on different sounds and what you could do to change or correct these errors. Using this information think what went wrong when you stuttered and now (5) review what you can do to slowly reverse or change the errors you made on this particular sound or word.

Next (6) mentally rehearse or pantomime how it would feel to slowly make these corrections so as to modify your usual pattern of stuttering and move through the word.

(As you take time to study your blocking problem and plan how to deal with it, it may seem to you that the person to whom you are talking may lose interest in what you have to say. That is possible but still you need to stick to your guns whenever you stutter and concentrate on working this post-block correction properly. Take your time as the pause needs to be long enough to accomplish your purpose of preparing your course of action.[1])

After you determine what you need to do to correct or modify the errors you made—and after you have mentally rehearsed how it will feel to say the word again while making these corrections—then and only then—(7) repeat the word as you feel yourself making the corrections.

BUT, this time (8) articulate the sound on which you blocked in a smooth flow prolonged resonant manner. This will give you time to concentrate on feeling your-

---

[1]As stutterers begin to put these pauses into their speech following their moments of stuttering while appearing relatively unruffled and unhurried, they find much more acceptance from those with whom they are communicating than they had expected. (Van-Riper)

self correcting or at least changing the speech muscle errors you made when you stuttered. And by keeping your voice flowing it will enable you to make the transition to the next sound more easily.[1]

In speaking in this way please remember to overcorrect your wrong speech muscle action. Change what you usually do when you block on a sound. For instance if it calls for a light contact press so lightly that there is little or no contact. And pay more attention to how the articulation of the words feels than how it sounds.

Although this post-block correction may seem to take a long time it should not take over a few seconds. The more you do it and become adept at it the less time it will take. You need to keep doing it when you stutter until you have become proficient at it.

The slow prolonged resonant way of working your way through the sound while keeping your voice flowing will give you plenty of time to feel yourself making the corrections you need to make. Of course you should not adopt this manner of talking generally—just use it in post-block corrections.

You need not be ashamed of repeating your stuttered words in this deliberate manner. The slight delay and the careful corrections will show others that you are determined to control your difficulty. Most listeners are considerate anyway but in this case they will actually respect you for your efforts.[2]

---

[1] Move slowly and gently from sound to sound through the word. (Neely)

[2] All of us respect a person who tries to cope with his disability even if he has trouble doing so. (VanRiper)

Persevere in using these corrections when you stutter. Their use will help you train yourself so you can move more easily through a block. They will break up the pattern of your stuttering and help you gain confidence in your ability to control your speech.

You will need plenty of opportunity to use post-block corrections and it may help some to practice them aloud when you are alone. It may not be necessary for you to spend more than a couple of weeks on this part of the program. But only when you feel that you have mastered this process should you proceed to the next step.

Pre-Block Correction

Presumably you have now conscientiously practiced and regularly employed post-block corrections when you stuttered. In doing this you learned new ways of responding and how to move through a block in a predetermined manner. You should now be adept at correcting your stuttering after it happens.

However, you may have felt that post-block corrections were like locking the barn door after the horse was stolen since the process did not stop the stuttering when it started. Of course you are right, but it is essential for you to have had this training because it paves the way for this seventh step. Now you need to learn how to make preparations to forestall your stuttering before it happens.[1] This process of controlling your blocks before they occur is called 'pre-block' correction.

Most of the time the stutterer anticipates when he may have trouble before it happens. In fact stuttering is sometimes referred to as an "anticipatory struggle reaction", which in effect says that the stutterer anticipates trouble and reacts by struggling to avoid it. Occasionally there is no anticipation and the blocks surprise you and this will be discussed later.

Since you usually have anticipation of difficulty before it happens we propose that you take advantage of this fact. To do so will give you an opportunity to respond to the threat of trouble by preparing for it ahead of time.

---

[1]You must learn how to prepare for the speech attempt on feared words so they can be spoken without interference or abnormality. (VanRiper)

So in this step it is suggested that you learn how to cope with your stuttering by moving out ahead of your block and approaching it in a new and better way through employing these pre-block corrections. They are similar to the post-block corrections except for the fact that your planning is done before (pre) rather than after (post) the need arises.

In the pre-block correction when you anticipate stuttering on a word or sound, you are to pause just before saying the word in order to plan how you will attack it. And you do not proceed to speak the word until you have thought about how you usually stutter on the sound and figure out what needs to be done to correct or modify the errors you usually make when stuttering on that sound.

Even though this course of action is similar to the post-block process, please study the following directions carefully so you will know exactly how it should be done. It is a key part of your therapy program.

To prevent any possible misunderstanding we outline in detail how these pre-block corrections should be put into action since it will require a lot of concentration on your part. The numbers in parenthesis refer to the steps in the procedure.

Pre-Block Correction—Sequence of Action

This is the exact procedure you should follow in using a pre-block correction when you approach a feared sound or word. Just as you come up to the word and before you start to say it, (1) pause—come to a complete stop. This pause before starting to say the word allows you time to calm yourself and to plan and rehearse how you will deal with the word.

This pause may cause some embarrassment,[1] but again you have got to have the courage to follow through on this. Others have done it; you can too. The pause will not be long and a willingness to halt will convince both you as well as your listener that you are determined to be in control of the situation.[2] Even if it takes longer the pause may be less embarrassing than your stuttering, particularly if you blunder into it blindly.

After you have stopped, the first thing you do is (2) try to relax the tensed area of your speech mechanism including your throat. Try to get that feeling of your tongue lying limp in the bottom of your mouth with your jaw slightly open as if you were going to drool with your lips loose. See if you can get a feeling of looseness in that area.

As you relax, think back and (3) recall what you usually do abnormally when you block on that sound. What errors do you usually make when you stutter on it? You should remember these errors from the analysis and study you made of your speech muscle activity in the fifth step and from your experience in making post-block corrections.

Then from this review of the errors you usually make (4) figure out what corrections you can put into effect to change what you usually do wrong when you stutter on that sound to help you remove or modify the abnormalities you make when you block on it.

---

[1]Stutterers fear silence almost as much as they do the exposure of their abnormality. (VanRiper)

[2]Society in general rewards the person who obviously confronts and attempts to deal with his stuttering. (Stromsta)

Then (5) rehearse in your mind, or actually panto-mime how it would feel to put these corrections into effect saying the whole word in a slow motion deliberate-ly prolonged manner, shifting slowly from one sound to the next. This means you are to mentally rehearse or pantomime how you will act out these changes to elimi-nate the errors you usually make on that sound.[1]

As your breathing returns to normal—and not be-fore—(6) say the word making the corrections as you rehearsed them. BUT (7) articulate the sound and word in a sliding resonant prolonged manner, exaggerating the corrections, paying more attention to how the word feels than how it sounds.[2] Although the slow articula-tion may carry over to the following few words you should not talk that way otherwise.

A problem is often encountered in making the tran-sition from the consonant sound to the vowel sound which follows. The slow prolonged manner of keeping the sounds flowing, as you utter the feared word, is de-signed to make that transition smooth.[3] Also it allows you sufficient time to get the feeling of making the cor-rections as you slide through the sound and word.[4] As

---

[1]First, he (the stutterer) is to reduplicate in pantomime a fore-shortened version of the stuttering behavior he has just experienced and, secondly, he is to rehearse again in pantomime, a modified ver-sion of that behavior. (VanRiper)

[2]Learn to be aware of the feeling of muscle action as you move through a word. (Neely)

[3]Any action that emphasizes or enhances smooth transitions from sound to sound, syllable to syllable, or word to word, will be beneficial for on-going speech. (Agnello)

[4]These corrected words may seem prolonged and drawling. That happens as a result of the more careful and slower movements you made while saying the word. These will speed up as your skill im-proves. We are not after slow drawling speech, but speech with more self-controlled movements. (Starbuck)

you move slowly through the word, concentrate on getting the feel of change or overcorrecting your abnormalities.

If you are embarrassed by the pause or by the drawling way you enunciate the feared word, do it anyway! This is where your determination pays off—you have no other choice. You will find that the pause will become shorter and shorter as you become more proficient at tackling your expected blocking in this new way.

> **Warning**—under no circumstances should you use the pause as a postponement, although it may be tempting to do so. The pause should be used to prepare and rehearse your plan of action.

This pre-block correction is an important part of your therapy program. If you can move smoothly through an anticipated block you are well on your way to speaking freely and fluently. Practice pre-block corrections on both feared and nonfeared words—or on the first word of a sentence[1] but do not use them as a trick to get started. Some stutterers have pre-blocked on every word while they were learning the technique but that should not be necessary. The effect of a good pre-block carries over.

Select words on which you might block—figure out how you usually stutter on them—then determine what changes you need to make and apply them when you get to the word. Whenever you suspect trouble, put your controls into effect and pre-block. Continue this practice until you automatically feel what corrections are required for any type of block. This should give you a great feeling of your stuttering being under control.

---

[1]It is always good to use a pre-block on the first word of a sentence. (Starbuck)

When you become so accustomed to using pre-block corrections that they are second nature to you, then you can start gradually eliminating the pause. When you anticipate trouble on a sound several words ahead, you can use the time during which you are saying the intervening words to prepare what you need to do when you reach the feared word.

Then put your speech into low gear (slow down) which will give you time to plan how you should make the necessary corrections. Then move slowly and smoothly through the word as you feel your way along.

This is your goal, and you may attain it fairly quickly, but until you have confidence in your ability to do it properly, it would be better for you first to stop and pause in order to allow yourself the time to make adequate preparations to deal with expected trouble.

As you get better at pre-block corrections you will be building confidence in your ability to control your speech so you can move through any block in a predetermined manner. You determine beforehand the movements you have to make and how you have to make them to form the sounds and say the words smoothly. It is important to follow through on this. Stuttering is something you do and you should now have learned how you can change what you have been doing.

In-Block Correction

With the post-block correction you learned how to cancel your stuttering after it occurred. With the pre-block correction you learned how you should act to prevent its occurrence. Now it is suggested that you use a comparable method of pulling out blocks of which you have had no advance warning.[1]

This is to be used in those instances when you stutter unexpectedly. Without the anticipatory fear build up, your tensions will not be as great but you still have a problem to resolve.[2] What do you usually do when you suddenly find yourself stuck in a block with no warning?

Perhaps you immediately try to escape from the block by using some intelligent procedure, but more probably you just struggle blindly, trying to force your way out, which only makes things worse, or you may resort to some release gimmick which has helped you in the past. We suggest that you try to use a systematic method, one that is compatible with this therapy approach.

To do this you should employ what is called an 'in-block' correction. Those stutterers who rarely anticipate difficulty will need to rely on this in-block correction more frequently than others but all stutterers may find is useful from time to time.

---

[1]You must learn how to pull out of your old blocks voluntarily, to get them under voluntary control before uttering the word. (Van-Riper)

[2]It is possible to release yourself voluntarily from blocking or repeating prior to completing a word utterance. (Czuchna)

The in-block correction will not stop your stuttering because you are already in trouble at the time you use it. But since you need to pull out of the predicament anyway, it is better to go about it in a predetermined manner. At least that makes better sense than just to struggle blindly.

Here's the way it works. When you find yourself in the middle of a block, don't pause and don't stop and try again. Instead, continue the stuttering, slowing it down and letting the block run its course, deliberately making a smooth prolongation of what you are doing.[1] In doing this you will be stabilizing the sound by slowing down a repetition, or changing the repetition to a prolongation, or smoothing out a tremor, or pulling out of a fixation as you ease out of the block.

In doing this you will come to realize that you can control the duration of your block by learning to smooth out your stutter.[2]

Anyway, hold the stuttering long enough to get control and to figure out what you are doing wrong, and what you need to do to reduce or eliminate the abnormality. From your previous study you should realize what you can do to counteract your faulty speech behavior.

After you have figured this out, then voluntarily release yourself by discontinuing the prolongation or repetions—and in slow motion put into effect the meas-

---

[1]He (the stutterer) can change the way he stutters by deliberately "hanging on to" or prolonging the troublesome sound without struggling or unnecessary forcing. (Luper)

[2]As stutterers learn that they can control the duration of the stuttering block, the fear of not being able to complete the message disappears. (D. Williams)

ures you decided would reverse or correct the abnormal speech muscle action.[1]

If for any reason you are unable to get hold of your stutter and move out of the block as described above, then it would be better for you to do a post-block correction in order for you to keep the feeling of being in control. In any case you should be able to correct what you did wrong because of what you have learned from your analysis and study of the way you stutter.

Even if you anticipate almost all of your stuttering, it may be a good idea to practice making in-block corrections since you may occasionally have to pull yourself out of a block. You can practice by faking blocks on both feared and non-feared words and then rehearsing your in-block corrections. It is better to have a planned approach for getting out of trouble and one that fits in with this program. Practicing on faked blocks isn't easy but can be of assistance.

It should not be necessary for you to use this in-block correction often, since usually you are aware of approaching trouble and can forestall it by pre-blocking, but you can use this technique when needed. With the training you have had, you should be able to react to warnings of approaching trouble. Remember if you suspect anything —pause—take your time—relax—plan properly—get set—and move through the feared word with a pre-block correction.

---

[1]In pulling out of blocks the stutterer does not let the original blocking run its course as he does in cancellation. Instead he makes a deliberate attempt to modify it before the release occurs and before the word is spoken. (VanRiper)

As a speech pathologist working with adult stutterers I have found that the most important factors that determine progress are (1) that the stutterer have a goal that requires better speech, and (2) that he form the habit of working consistently and steadily to accomplish his purpose. Someone once told me that the price of better speech is keeping steadily at it. (Gregory)

Review—Follow Through

After you have become adept at using the block corrections, you have completed the steps in this program. But there are still a few things to do and think about. First, let's review what we hope you have accomplished. At the beginning we suggested that you conform to nine common sense ground rules which are conducive to better speech.

Now would be a good time to review these ground rules which are listed on page 33 to see if your speech is still being guided by these recommendations. Have you tried to live up to these rules?

Then you started on the other steps in therapy. First we wanted you to willingly admit to others that you were a stutterer. Designed to reduce your sensitivity, this admission—including voluntary stuttering—should have helped reduce your anxiety and fear. Have you done this?

Next you were called on to eliminate your secondary symptoms, the abnormal, unattractive or useless habits which you had acquired as accessory behaviors to your stuttering. These movements had probably become part of your stuttering pattern but had nothing to do with the production of speech. Have you gotten rid of them?

Following this you were asked to stop all your avoidance and postponement habits, since they only gave temporary relief, and only built up and sustained your anxieties. It is vitally important for you to have eliminated such habits. We hope you don't avoid or postpone any more. Honestly, have you dropped all such practices?

Next you were to habitually maintain eye contact with those to whom you talked to help combat feelings of inadequacy or embarrassment. Do you now keep eye contact when stuttering?

If you conscientiously completed these four steps you became what is called an "honest" stutterer without any accessory or unnecessary frills. Accordingly, your stuttering was then confined to irregularities in the way you operated your speech mechanism. You were then asked to attack any remaining abnormal speech muscle activity.

Since practically all stutterers have only a vague idea of what their speech mechanism does when they stutter, you were then instructed to find out what you did abnormally with your speech muscles if or when you blocked.

This called for a close study of your stuttering and if you followed the assignments carefully you figured out how you could talk differently by either eliminating unnecessary movements or by making changes in your particular pattern. Habits which have been learned can be unlearned.

Then in the next step you practiced using post-block corrections after you stuttered. These corrections were planned and organized to help you to relax your tension and to eliminate or modify the speech muscle errors you made when stuttering. They were designed to help you guide your speech muscle movements so you could move easily and smoothly into, through and out of your blocks by substituting new patterns for old habits. Did you follow through?

Finally you learned how to forestall trouble by putting into effect pre-block corrections which worked on the same principle. Taking advantage of the fact that you usually anticipate when you will stutter, you responded by getting set and making preparatory moves to change or contradict the abnormal speech activity which characterized your blocks.

This, of course, was a key procedure and its description was outlined in detail. Then it was explained how to use a compatible procedure to pull out of trouble when you had a block of which you had no advance warning.

In Conclusion

If you have done all these things, in a sense you have completed this therapy program. We don't know how fluent you have become—possibly you have come a long way—possibly you haven't. This book only describes an approach which will work. You are the one who has produced the results.[1]

In this program, if you have learned nothing else, you should have found out that you can change your way of talking.[2] That's for sure. And if you can learn to change your way of talking, you can control your stuttering. You want and need that feeling of control which enables you to talk smoothly and comfortably.

And if you stuck to your guns in this program we'll bet you're glad that you didn't back out. But even for those who have made rapid progress we advise caution.

---

[1]It is not a matter of luck. You can make your own "luck". You can get there. (J. D. Williams)

[2]By learning that he has a choice in the way he talks and in the manner in which he reacts, he will come to realize that he can be responsible for the way he talks. He will come to be the kind of speaker who can change the speaking he does. (D. Williams)

Strange as it may seem you may need to adjust to fluent speech.

You may need to monitor your speech as you become fluent, depending on your reactions. For instance you might start talking so fast that you do not become aware of avoidances or struggles that could develop. Furthermore, since you have not been used to talking freely, any inability to express yourself in managing phrases or sentences may cause you to lose confidence in your way of talking, etc.

Unfortunately, stuttering seems to be particularly susceptible to reoccurring.[1] You will need to guard against slipping back into old habits. Habits which you acquired years ago and which have been performed for many years can reinstate themselves if you aren't careful. You could at times be confronted with old fears.

If you should be confronted with such fears, the most important point for you to remember is that a willingness to stutter in a modified way can be a tremendous factor toward sustaining and reinforcing your fluency.

Also to help prevent backsliding or regression be careful and do your best to make certain that your speech is governed so that you talk in accordance with the ground rules. These common sense measures can always help you communicate with less stress and strain. And be sure that you do not start avoiding.

If you should run into any usual difficulty you can always use your block controls. It might be well to review and practice them occasionally anyway, since you may always be able to use them to advantage.

---

[1]Traces of the disorder usually remain and relapses occur. (Freund)

Actually as time passes on, you should continue to gain confidence in your ability to control your speech.[1] And the more success you have, the more freedom from fear you will experience.

On the other hand don't expect or claim too much.[2] Don't be too anxious to talk too well too soon and don't make excessive demands on your speech which will be impossible to achieve. And don't be fooled into thinking that just because you don't stutter that that automatically makes you witty, charming and persuasive.[3]

If someone says you are cured, don't feel that you have to prove it. Instead tell him or her that you still stutter and actually show them that you can do so by stuttering voluntarily. If you always call yourself a stutterer you will be under no pressure not to be one. Remember stuttering is largely what the stutterer does trying not to stutter.

Your speech, like others, doesn't have to be perfect.[4] Most people are disfluent. No one—and we mean no one —has verbal perfection—ex-stutterers or not. Stuttering is a stubborn handicap and if you have conquered it

---

[1]Confidence comes when we do battle and succeed. It comes when we accept a challenge instead of running away from it. (Van-Riper)

[2]On the whole people who stutter are highly intelligent and capable. Yet there appears to be a discrepancy between their realistic capabilities and what they realistically expect of themselves . . . To avoid this dilemma, make your expectations more reasonable. (Barbara)

[3]Stutterers are no better or no worse than anyone else, and you would not necessarily set the world on fire if you only did not stutter. You would just talk better. (Emerick)

[4]Perfect fluency is not obtainable and is a self-defeating goal. (Sheehan)

to the extent that you have freedom from fear, you can no longer claim it as a handicap. Therapy is a challenge as life is a challenge. Have faith in yourself.[1]

And if you have just been reading this book for information, we would again point out that there is no reason for you to spend the rest of your life stuttering helplessly and making yourself miserable. Others have prevailed and so can you.

The End

---

[1]After all, fellow stutterers, there are strength and resources within each of us. Only through these can we really accomplish anything. (Brown)

I am a stutterer. I am not like other people. I must think differently, act differently, live differently—because I stutter. Like other stutterers, like other exiles, I have known all my life a great sorrow and a great hope together, and they have made me the kind of person I am. An awkward tongue has molded my life. (Johnson)

Appendix

HOW TO WORK ON

Eliminating Secondary Symptoms

In this step you examine your speech to find out what secondary symptoms you might have (if any) and make a list of them.[1] This refers to any unnatural movement or mannerism you might exhibit when stuttering, although it does not refer to any abnormal activity of the speech mechanism itself.

There is no universal secondary symptom which is common to all stutterers. You may blink your eyes, swing your arm, protrude your lip, jingle your coins or blow your nose, etc. It could be anything. The problems discussed in this chapter may be different from yours, but that is not important since they are just used as examples and the principles of correction outlined will apply to any stuttering habit or trick.

The difficult part of the problem is how to get rid of a secondary symptom. Start out by selecting just one to attack since it is better to work on one at a time. Perhaps it is a tough one.[2] Many are.

To work on eliminating it you must first become aware of the behavior at the moment it happens. You have to be alert to do this because any such movement is usually automatic and involuntary and often you do not fully realize what it is and when you are doing it.

---

[1]Make an inventory of speech related struggle that accompanies your stuttering. (Moses)

[2]Another philosophy of my therapy has been that by tackling situations of greater difficulty, others that were once hard become easier. (Gregory)

As an example you might be interested in how one stutterer eliminated a rather grotesque secondary symptom of head jerking. This is how he told it.

"I'd always hated my head jerking. Looked awful, I know, and it bothered other people but I'd never been able to control it until now. It just seemed to take off when I blocked hard. I suffered from it for many years but it's gone now. I've learned how to keep it out and now my fear of stuttering has gone way down and I'm not stuttering much.

"Here's how I did it. It was suggested that I watch myself in the mirror when making phone calls. At first I could not bear to look at my jerking in the mirror but kept at it and finally got curious about it. So I studied it. I found that I jerked it suddenly and always to the right side. It occurred only after I tensed my jaw and neck greatly and only after a series of fast repetitions. Why did I always have to let it jerk to the right? What happened just before the jerk? I noticed that I also squinted one eye (the right one) just before it happened. I found that on my easier blockings my eye didn't squint.

"Well, then I began to change these things.[1] I made more phone calls and tried to jerk my head in the same way but on words I wasn't afraid of, and more slowly and on purpose. Then when the real head-jerking occurred, I tried jerking it to the left or moving my head and jaw slowly rather than swiftly. I found I could

---

[1]Set up a program of change. Take all the different elements that make up your stuttering pattern, e.g. head jerks, eye blinks, etc. Then consciously and deliberately attempt to add (exaggerate), vary (instead of jerking your head to the right, jerk it to the left) and drop out the separate parts one at a time. Break up the stereotyped nature of how you go about doing your stuttering. (Emerick)

change and control it and when I did, I didn't feel help-less. I got so I could change the involuntary jerk into a voluntary one.

"Then I was no longer a slave to the habit but the master. Also by slowing down the repetitions, that pre-ceded it I discovered that I could prevent it from hap-pening. There was one other thing that I did too that helped greatly. I experimented with relaxing my jaw and neck when beginning to stutter. Couldn't always do it, but when I did I found I could keep my head steady and in control. What a relief! I've got a long ways to go but at least when I stutter I'm no longer that abnormal monster I once was."

Another stutterer had a habit of tapping his foot when he stuttered, sort of beating time to the word or syllable.[1] To find out how bad it was and exactly what he was doing, the suggestion was made that he pick out some speaking situations and count the number of times he tapped his foot when stuttering. It was most difficult for him to do this, but he finally was able to get a count and discovered that they usually came on certain words or sounds when he was under stress.

Then he experimented with over-tapping more than he ordinarily would. He also practiced tapping purposely when he did not stutter, although he had to be partic-ularly careful to be sure it was done voluntarily. The

---

[1]To me syllable-tapping was an old story that had no happy ending. I had tried it in junior high and high school, using an ordi-nary lead pencil. Vividly I recall my embarrassment when I pressed too hard and the pencil lead flew high in the air, to everyone's amusement but mine. After that I tapped for awhile on the eraser end, then gave it up completely, so I thought. But finger-tapping re-mained a part of my instrumental stuttering pattern for many en-suing years. (Sheehan)

idea, of course, was to bring his compulsive tapping under conscious control. Then he worked on varying the way he tapped when he was stuttering by doing it differently than he ordinarily would. He would plan ahead of time how he would vary it so that he could have the feeling of it being under his control.

Do you get the idea? In order to work on eliminating a secondary symptom it is important to investigate it down to the smallest detail, since you need to understand what you are doing before you can expect to win the battle against any such habit.[1] As you gain this knowledge then you should start to vary your behavior. It is always helpful to purposely act out your symptom (whatever it may be) when you are not stuttering.

The key to eliminating it is to get it under conscious control from an involuntary movement to a voluntary movement. If you forget and find that you are not in control then start over again. As you talk, voluntarily vary the way you do it on purpose. Practice taking over control in anxiety producing situations until you know you are the master and can skip it altogether.

The basic idea is to make the behavior voluntary while it is occurring—then to vary it voluntarily—then to curtail its duration—then to stutter on the word without it. You can stop these mannerisms if you are determined to do so.

---

[1]The mannerism should be closely observed in the mirror, studied, analyzed, imitated, practiced and deliberately modified. (Johnson)

HOW TO WORK ON

Eliminating Avoidances, Substitutions and Postponements

Naturally your first assignment in this step is to find out how often and under what circumstances you avoid, substitute or postpone. We could cite examples of what other stutterers do, but the real test must come from self-observation. You need to find out what you do and how you avoid so you will know what needs to be changed. And then it may pretty well boil down to how much determination you have.

Start to observe your actions or lack of action and make memorandums of what you find. Avoidances are of most importance but postponements and substitutions are often involved and cover a lot of ground. So study your reactions and make notes of what you do or don't do.[1]

Why shouldn't you avoid answering the phone when someone else can do so? Or why shouldn't you substitute easier said words for those on which you have difficulty? There is one good reason—and it is a powerful one. The more you make a practice of avoiding, postponing and substituting, the more you will reinforce your fear of

---

[1]Make a list of all your avoidances: What types do you use (starters, delaying tactics, etc.)? When, in what contexts do you use them? How frequently do you resort to evasion? In other words, prepare an avoidance inventory. Then, systematically vary and exaggerate each one; use the avoidances when you don't need to in a highly voluntary manner. Finally, when you find yourself using an avoidance involuntarily, invoke a self-penalty; for example, if you avoid the word "chocolate," you must then use that word several times immediately thereafter. One of the best penalties is to explain to the listener the avoidance you have just used and why you should resist such evasions. (Emerick)

stuttering. Why keep building up more fear? If there is one thing the stutterer needs more than anything else it is to reduce his fears and certainly not reinforce them.[1]

And the less you avoid the more confidence you will have in yourself as a respectable and worthy person. That doesn't mean that you need to go overboard as we said before and immediately begin to make speeches before an audience, but in the give and take of normal life, you should not back down but speak up. To come right out and stutter openly will take courage on your part. Sure, it is miserable to stutter openly but in order to conquer your stuttering you must not be afraid to stutter. You have been running away too long. Now is a good time to stand and fight.[2]

Did the phone just now ring? Don't push others away so you can answer it, but if you would normally be the logical person to take the call, do so. That may be tackling your biggest bugaboo. Perhaps you say to yourself that it's too much and you just can't do it. Possibly you should tackle easier objectives first. That's a matter of judgment, but even if you are not trying to overcome your stuttering, you can not expect to go through life always avoiding the telephone. Sooner or later you'll have to take up that receiver and talk, and the longer you

---

[1]What happens is this: The successful avoidance causes some anxiety reduction. Then, when a similar situation presents itself, the need to avoid is even stronger due to the preceding reinforcement. But now, no avoidance is possible. The conflict becomes even greater. And so several vicious circles (or rather spirals) are set into motion. (VanRiper)

[2]The habitual avoidance of speaking situations and feared words will get you nowhere in the long run. (Murray)

put it off, the harder it will be. A large part of your stuttering abnormality comes from avoidances so start whittling them away.

On the other hand possibly it doesn't particularly bother you to talk on the phone but you have other problems. Let's assume that you did answer that call just now when the phone rang and you talked to the person at the other end of the line. During the conversation did you come to a word on which you expected to stutter and then did you think of another way of saying it to avoid trouble on that word? Possibly you did. If so, you added another brick to the wall of your fear.

It is difficult to observe yourself but resolve the next time you talk you will not substitute words.[1] You sure are going to have to watch yourself carefully because you may be doing that all the time. Say what you have to say and if you stutter, so what? You've stuttered before and it didn't kill you.

Incidentally when you saw so-and-so the other day and you were afraid you might stutter if you had to talk to him, what did you do? How did you get around speaking to him? Did you cross to the other side of the room or did you hide from him—or did you just clam up? Unfortunately we do not know what sort of contacts or meetings you avoid, but you do!

As you have had the habit of planning how you could avoid trouble, now spend time planning how not to avoid trouble. At times you may fail to follow through but if you do, you should make up for such failures by entering

---

[1]The author knows from his own past experience as a severe stutterer and from his dealings with many other stutterers, that it is better to have a five-minute blocking than to avoid a word successfully. We never conquer fear by running away; we only increase it. (VanRiper)

other or similar situations in which you are afraid you might stutter.[1] No one wins all the time but one can always recoup. In any case be honest with yourself regarding any such assignments. If you alibi you are kidding no one but yourself.

As we said before when you run into normal situations when you would like to talk, make a point of taking advantage of them and speak up.[2] Your opinions need to be heard as well as those of the next person and use whatever words that come to you. Plan to express your thoughts without making substitutions or revisions to avoid stuttering.[3] If you have the determination to tackle your problems in this way, you will build confidence in yourself and it will make you happier.

Here's an account of what one stutterer did in trying to reduce the avoidances that constantly reinforced his fears, as he tells it.

"For years I've been using every imaginable trick I could think of to keep from stuttering or to hide it when it came. Most of the time I can get away with it, but even so I live with the fear that sooner or later I will be unmasked and I usually am. But the worst of it is the constant vigilance I've got to keep, the constant sizing up of situations and sentences for signs of approaching trouble. It's like walking through a jungle alone. And I get so tired of always having to get ready to duck and dodge and cover up this constant fear.

---

[1]Deliberately enter previously feared situations. (Moses)

[2]One way of reducing your fear is by increasing the amount of speaking you do, particularly in situations that you customarily avoid. (Trotter)

[3]Search for those words and situations that are beginning to bug you rather than hiding them until they build up giant fears. (Luper)

"Anyway today, thoroughly fed up, I decided to attack the situation head-on. I began by going to a cafe for breakfast rather than the cafeteria where I've always gone so I wouldn't have to talk. I walked past the cafe three times before getting up enough courage to walk in, but I finally did.

"I found myself rehearsing my order, changing my selections so I might not stutter, but I was so disgusted with my weakness that when the waitress came I just blurted out "b-b-b-bacon and eggs!" and stuttered on purpose on bacon. I looked at her and she didn't bat an eye. Just asked me if I wanted coffee and I said again "b-b-b-bacon and eggs and coffee." I can't tell you how good I felt. For once I hadn't been a coward. If they don't like it, they can lump it! I felt strong, not weak and I sure enjoyed the bacon and eggs.

"After breakfast I was feeling so good about myself that I decided to tackle the phone which has always been my most feared situation. I wanted to find out when the buses left for Trenton, and ordinarily I might have gone to the bus station rather than phone. That phone fear is terrible and I hung up twice when they answered before saying a word. I was in such a panic I hardly knew what I wanted to say even if I could have started.

"So I sat down, smoked a cigarette, and wrote out the words "When do the buses leave for Trenton this afternoon?" put the mirror by the phone so I could see myself, dialed the number and then said it word by word. I stuttered though not as much as I'd expected, and I had to say it twice because the clerk didn't understand the first time but I got the information I needed. Felt all drained out afterwards but also triumphant. I'll lick this damned thing yet!"

So can you.

HOW TO WORK ON

Maintaining Eye Contact

This may represent more of a problem than you think. Perhaps you have become so shy that it is difficult for you to look at anybody when you are stuttering. It is suggested that you double-check yourself carefully and try the following procedures.

Start by looking at yourself in the mirror when alone and faking an easy block. Do you keep eye contact with yourself or do you avert your eyes? Try this repeatedly making sure that you don't look away. That shouldn't be too hard. Then do it when making a severe block. If you find you do not keep eye contact before and during the block, work at it until you find that you can and continue doing it.

Then make some phone calls looking at yourself in the mirror while you are having real blocks. Watch yourself until you can talk without shifting your eyes during five or more real stutterings.[1] As one stutterer remarked, "It ain't easy," but to complete this program successfully is a necessary step.

As you become more sure of yourself it will be easier for you to maintain eye contact while talking in general conversation.[2] This does not require that you stare fixidly or glare at your listener but look at him in a normal natural way.

---

[1] Read a sentence, look up into the mirror, paraphrase the sentence while maintaining eye contact. (Adler)

[2] Be sure you don't look down or away at the moment of stuttering. Some people will look away no matter how much you try to keep contact. To succeed it is sufficient that you look at them. (Sheehan)

While talking to others collect one, two, and then three occasions in which you maintain good contact when and as you are stuttering. Then make it ten occasions. As some evidence that you have followed through, it is suggested you write down the names and eye colors of ten people to whom you have stuttered.

Use your ingenuity in devising other pertinent assignments. Build confidence in your ability to speak with good natural eye contact on all occasions from now on, and you will feel better for doing so. It will give you satisfaction to know that you can clear another hurdle in making progress toward your goal.

Melinda didn't have this problem.[1]

---

[1] Melinda always maintained excellent eye contact. She had beautiful jet black eyes, and she kept them upon you constantly, testing, testing, testing. The intensity of her gaze increased at the moments of her stuttering. At the same time, however, she smiled, a bitter sweet smile. Not much humor in it—just a beautiful, brave girl smiling away the monsters and the ghosts. (VanRiper)

HOW TO WORK ON

Analyzing Blocks

In this step you are asked to examine yourself to find out what you are doing with your speech muscles when you stutter.[1] There is no way for us to know what happens in your case. But we list here some probabilities or variations of stuttering behavior which may happen with you when uttering a sample consonant sound. This may give you a better idea of what you may discover.

It should first be explained that all vocal expression or speech is actually made up of separate and different sounds which are combined to make words.[2] To express it in another way, when you talk you articulate sounds which form words. In the interest of simplicity these sounds will be referred to as vowel and consonant sounds —the vowel sounds being A, E, I, etc., and the consonant sounds B, C, D, etc.

When you stutter you may think that you are blocking on a word. You are right, but more specifically you are blocking on a sound of that word or on making the transition from one sound to the next. To use a simple illustration when you stutter saying b-b-b-ball you are not blocking on the word "ball" but on the consonant sound 'B' or on the transition from 'B' to 'A'. Most stutterers find their greatest difficulty in shifting from one sound to the next in order to produce the necessary syllable.

---

[1]You've got to examine and analyze the act of speaking to see what errors you are making. (Starbuck)

[2]You may think of a word as being a unit or lump of sound. Actually a word is composed of separate sounds much as a written word consists of separate letters. (Neely)

Among other possibilities you may find out that your airflow is sporadic or jerky; or you let all your air out first and then try to talk without sufficient breath; or you use some kind of starter noises or interjections; or you jam your lips shut and can't get them apart; or your tongue sticks to the roof of your mouth; or you have rapid-fire repetitions or just repeat sounds; or you have tremors in your jaw; or you have prolongation of certain sounds, etc.

It would be impossible to describe how to correct all kinds of faulty speech behavior. To attempt such an explanation would involve too many complicated procedures exceedingly difficult to explain in writing even if we did know what happens in your case.

However, let's try out your speech muscle activity on a sample consonant sound. For lack of a better example, let's assume that your name is Peter and you have particular trouble with the 'P' sound and the transition to the next sound.

(Virtually every stutterer has trouble with his own name, particularly when he is called on to identify himself to someone in authority.)

For your information the 'P' sound is called a "labial plosive." This kind of sound is correctly made by closing your lips and building up slight air pressure and then suddenly releasing the air by separating your lips quickly.

Anyway, now in front of your mirror, stutter badly on the 'P' sound as you say your name putting as much tension into it as you usually do. Then stutter on it again in the same way but this time do it in extremely slow motion so you can have an opportunity for feeling what your speech muscles are doing while you block. Repeat this several times.

What happened and what did you find out? Certainly you had an excessive amount of tension but where was it principally located? Perhaps there was no passage of air because your tight lips closed the airway. Or maybe you tried to say the name without sufficient breath, or your airflow was obstructed by your tongue. Stutterers do that sometimes. Obviously, you can't talk without breath flow. Or perhaps you shut off the airflow in your throat by tightening your vocal cords excessively.

Some therapists believe that the key to therapy is an airflow technique. They claim that if breath is gently and passively initiated and flowing just prior to speech it will enable the stutterer to avoid trouble.

This is somewhat similar to the reasoning behind the "sigh" technique which was in vogue many years ago. That principle stated that if the stutterer made a slight sigh as he tackled a block it would keep the vocal cords open and relaxed and enable him to move through the block without trouble.

This technique works at first but after the distraction effect wears off, the stutterer is usually left with breathing abnormalities including speaking on the end of the breath, gasping and hyperventilation with a resulting increase in tension. One of the problems in therapy is to synchronize breathing, voice and articulation in the utterance of a sound.

When the timing is broken and needs to be unified, concentration on just one of these features can ruin the coordination.

But don't be afraid to experiment. Find a way to keep the speech airways open. A normal speaker initiates airflow simultaneously with the speech attempt.[1] Research has shown that in normal utterance the breath flow does not begin before the person assumes the articulatory posture but occurs simultaneously.

Perhaps instead of attacking the 'P' sound directly, you hemmed and hawed, using various repetitive starter sounds like 'uh' or 'er' or 'well', etc. Or maybe you stopped and started again repeating a phrase. Because of the tension your speech muscles may have become temporarily frozen in a rigid position thus blocking any sound.

Possibly you had tiny vibrations in your lips or jaw— or possibly the sound came out p-p-p-p repetitively in sort of a bounce pattern like a broken record. Or maybe your lips were squeezed or protruded and set in a fast vibration or trembling called a tremor.

Much more likely you blocked because you held your mouth in a fixed position. In other words you pressed your lips together so tightly on the 'P' sound that you couldn't separate them and let the air escape. You couldn't uncork your mouth because you were making such a hard tight contact. Are you doing these things?

Of course you are not doing all these things and running into all these complications, but you need to write down how and where you get blocked making the 'P' sound. You will need this list to use as a reminder of what should be eliminated or modified.

---

[1]Breath control is best when it is automatic and not under conscious control . . . Breathing should be relatively automatic and unconscious so, in general, the less attention you give to it, the better. (Luper)

Now still in front of your mirror say your name *without* stuttering, in extremely slow motion repeatedly to get the feel of the difference between how you stutter and how you say it without stuttering.

In the latter case you will observe your tension is low and that you attack the word or sound without any starter sounds or interjections. Also when speaking normally, you don't repeat anything so there's no stopping and starting—no retrials. You have no vibrations or tremors in your lips or jaw—nor do you press or jam your lips together so hard that you cannot separate them. Feel the difference.

Anyway, let's make the assumption that your difficulty with the 'P' sound occurred because you pressed or squeezed your lips together so tightly or firmly that the sound was blocked. What can or should you do to change or correct that habit?

You can correct it by relaxing the tension in your lips and controlling them in order to keep the pressure from building up. When you start to say your name relax your lips so they feel weak and flabby—and then consciously control their movement so that they come together only very slightly as you utter the 'P' sound.[1] This is called a 'light contact.'

To produce a light contact you have to control the action of your lip muscles so that they just barely touch with no pressure whatsoever.[2] In this way you can consciously control the action of your lips so that they touch

---

[1]Concentrate on controlling the lip muscles so that they just barely touch and air is able to flow between them. (Starbuck)

[2]We must enable them to learn that it is possible to start a feared P word, for example, without pressing the lips together with compulsive force. (VanRiper)

only lightly as you allow the air from your breath to flow between them.[1] Practice making light loose contacts so you can get the feel of maneuvering your lip movement through the 'P' sound.

Using this as an example you should try to figure out how you can control your speech muscle action on other sounds in order to correct or change other bad speech habits that you may have acquired. Many of them are fairly simple to understand and can be modified and corrected through the application of other corrective procedures.[2]

Others are more complex but if you analyze your faulty speech habits carefully, it is reasonable to expect that you should be able to use controls which will modify or eliminate your unnatural or unnecessary actions.[3]

The more you continue to study the way you stutter on the sounds and words on which you have difficulty and then compare them with your fluent speech, the more you will realize that there is no reason you should not be able to move through a block easily without struggling. There is no need for you to spend the rest of your life struggling with blocks and making yourself miserable. Have faith in your ability to conquer your problem.

---

[1] As you say an isolated word beginning with a B or P for example, concentrate on the feeling of movement as you bring your lips together and as they move to the next sound. (Neely)

[2] You, too, can explore the unknown. When you do you may find that you push your lips too hard or jam your tongue against the roof of your mouth. (Luper)

[3] The better your understanding of your speech problem, and of what you are doing to complicate the problem, the more you can do to help yourself feel capable of dealing with it successfully. (Johnson)

Explaining to a Non-Stutterer the
Effect of Fear

If you should have occasion to explain to a non-stutterer how fear of difficulty can affect one's speech, the following illustration could be used. Assuming the non-stutterer has nothing wrong with his legs, you would point out that he should be able to walk easily without trouble or "fluently" along a long plank, twelve inches wide, when it is placed on the ground.

But if that same plank were situated on a brick wall high off the ground, then he would become apprehensive and develop a fear of falling if he were asked to walk along the plank at such height. As a result, even if he could force himself to walk the length of the plank, he would probably put on a poor exhibition of smooth or "fluent" walking.

This example is somewhat parallel to your problem as a stutterer. You have the physical equipment to talk properly, but have a fear of speech difficulty (developed from past experiences) which causes you to try to force trouble-free speech. And since smooth speech cannot be forced the result is that you do not speak "fluently."

Relevant and Interesting Quotations

Relevant and
Interesting Quotations

The quotations in this section were not written as answers to any of the questions asked, but do represent enlightened educational comments on the topics specified.

Is stuttering inherited?

There is no organic proof of stuttering being inherited, although we do know there is a familial tendency. Stuttering does run in families more often than in those of non-stutterers. Studies have found that over 65 percent of patients who stutter show a family history of stuttering. (Barbara)

Are there many stutterers?

Few realize that almost one percent of the population stutter, that there are more than a million and a half stutterers in the United States today. That many famous people from history have had essentially the same problem, including Moses, Demosthenes, Charles Lamb, Charles Darwin, and Charles I of England. More recently, George VI of England, Somerset Maugham, Marilyn Monroe, and the T. V. personalities, Garry Moore and Jack Paar have been stutterers at some time in their lives. In your speech problem you may not be as unique or as much alone as you had thought! (Sheehan)

The incidence of stuttering amounts to about 1,500,000 in this country alone, 15,000,000 in the world. It has been placed at about one percent of the general population, roughly half of them are children. Stuttering has no respect for social or economic status, religion, race or intelligence.

The problem of stuttering was recorded by the ancients. Aristotle, Hippocrates, Galen, and Celsus all theorized about the causes of stuttering and proposed remedies for its cure, among them the use of healing oils, cauterization of the tongue, and breathing exercises. World famous figures who were stutterers included Moses, Aristotle, Aesop, Demosthenes, Virgil, Charles I, Charles Lamb, Charles Darwin, and in modern times, Sir Winston Churchill, W. Somerset Maugham, and George VI. (Barbara)

Does stuttering vary?

No two stutterers perform their stuttering in exactly the same way, and any one stutterer varies somewhat in manner of performance during any given day, or hour, and from week to week and from year to year. (Barbara)

———

The frequency and severity of stuttering usually varies with the amount of communicative stress. Most stutterers speak fluently when alone or talking to pets or when reading in unison. A few do not. A few even stutter when they sing.

Stuttering is intermittent. Even severe stutterers often speak more words normally than in stuttered fashion. Only one of our cases, a neurotic hysterical girl whose disorder had its onset in an emotional upheaval at nineteen, stuttered consistently on every word, big or little, and even she would occasionally forget and speak fluently. The intermittency, however, makes the experience more distressful, since it is difficult to adapt to unpleasantness which comes and goes. (VanRiper)

Is the stutterer handicapped?

Your major handicap stems from the fact that you labor under the illusion that you are a handicapped person, because you believe that your stuttering is not your personal responsibility, that it is something that happens to you rather than something you do yourself. (Johnson)

Shouldn't the stutterer try to relax?

I have found that instruction in progressive and differential muscle relaxation is valuable in helping the stutterer to reduce tension during speech. Also the stutterer's thinking of, and striving for relaxation when under stress seems to have the effect of bringing about a general relaxation of his anxiety.

I continue to learn. I have practiced relaxation procedures as one approach to modifying the muscular tension involved in stuttering and to diminishing emotional arousal during speaking. Relaxation has been generally useful when I have needed to be more calm during a crisis.   (Gregory)

What are secondary symptoms like?

With stammering, there are countless manifestations of the speech struggle. The early symptoms may be nothing more than twitching of the face, blinking of the eyelids, or jerking of the head. With one patient there was elevation of an eyebrow, and sometimes of both eyebrows. Another patient would retract the right corner of the mouth when he began to stammer. Still another patient would protrude the tongue; he said that the tongue got stiff, then he got stiff all over. With severe stammering the jaw and head may participate in the contortion. The patient opens the mouth wider and wider with successive jerking movements, then throws the head violently backward. The arms and legs may engage in the struggle. The patient may clench the hands; he may jerk the arms; he may stamp a foot; he may writhe and twist his body.   (Bluemel)

When does a stutterer stutter?

When the stutterer's morale or ego strength is high because of achievements, success or social acceptance, he will tend to stutter less. If in any given communicative situation he expects or feels communicative stress, penalties, and frustrations he will stutter more.

He will stutter more if he is experiencing or anticipating anxiety, guilt and hostility. He will also stutter more if in scanning ahead he sees words or situations coming which have been associated with past experiences or stuttering.

Stutterers have more trouble talking to authority figures, to people who have become impatient or mock or suffer when listening to stuttering. Most stutterers are very vulnerable to listener loss, to interruptions, to rejections, penalty, frustration, anxiety and hostility.

The pressures then, which create more stuttering can come from within or without, from the pressures of the present, the expected agonies of the future or the miseries of the past. (VanRiper)

What part does fear play?

All of which is a way of saying that there is no stuttering where there is no fear of stuttering. (Johnson)

_____

Word and situation fears develop most readily when frequent difficulty is experienced on the same word or in the same situation and when the individual is very aware of having difficulty. (Luper)

_____

Once stuttering creates fear, and this fear, more fear and more stuttering, the disorder can exist on a self-sustaining basis. It can maintain and perpetuate itself even though the original causes may long since have lost all effectiveness and importance. Predisposing or precipitating causes have little importance, once the chain reaction gets going. (VanRiper)

_____

It is of vital importance for the stutterer to become thoroughly familiar with the emotional aspects of his affliction, for it is in this realm of behavior that he is finding difficulty in facing social situations where speech is required. Not only is the tension exhibited in the organs of speech a needless and futile struggle, but just as unreasonable are the sham battles going on within the emotional life of the stutterer, warping his perception of reality, blinding his vision with fear, blocking the potential expression of his personality, and binding him to the mast of inferiority. (Wedburg)

Shouldn't the stutterer take responsibility for his problem?

I also found, in working on my speech, that one makes many discoveries that can be applied advantageously to daily living. From the time I began therapy I have realized that I must take responsibility for my behavior and the way in which others evaluate me. In addition, I became aware of the tendency to lean on my stuttering as an excuse for not participating in some activity or for not being as successful as I might strive to be. (Gregory)

Is it hard to pause while talking?

Many stutterers show a *fear of silence* and any momentary pause or cessation of sound in their own speech brings on reactions approaching panic. Perhaps because most stuttering occurs on initial syllables and the stutterer has more trouble when he starts, he learns to dread the necessity for starting. He learns to dread any period of silence in his own speech, to fear it, and to become quite intolerant of it. (Sheehan)

Shouldn't one speak up?

Since speaking is a healthy and volitional form of self-expression, the stutterer should encourage himself to "speak up" and "speak with others," not as a performance task, but as a means of arriving at social communion and communication. At first this will appear embarrassing and difficult, but the more you accept your shortcomings and the less you put emphasis on your impediment, the more relaxed you will become and the greater interest will you develop in self-expression.   (Barbara)

Shouldn't one be less sensitive?

During my first two years in college I began to see more clearly that a stutterer has to take responsibility for making others feel comfortable in his presence. If he can be less sensitive about his stuttering those around him will be more comfortable, this will make him more at ease, he will stutter less, and so it goes; the vicious circle will be put into reverse. Since I was doing something constructive about my speech, I could smile about difficulty more. I could even feign some voluntary disfluency.   (Gregory)

What is there to worry about?

My youth, as is the case with so many stutterers, was filled with alternate hope and despair as I hungered for some relief from my stuttering. This of course is not unique; most stutterers have had similar feelings. But have you ever asked yourself what it is that really bothers you, what it is that causes despair? Is it your stuttering or is it your fear of people's reactions to your stuttering? Isn't it the latter? Most stutterers have too much anxiety about what they think people might say or do as a result of the stuttering.

These anxieties can be lessened.

I remember well these feelings of worry, anxiety, and despair. If you can learn to dissipate some of these terrible feelings—you will be able to help yourself as many other stutterers have done.

There is one effective method you can utilize to achieve this goal. Face your fears! This advice is easy to give and admittedly difficult for many of you to take; however, it is advice that has helped many stutterers and it can help you.

Somehow you must learn to desensitize yourself to the reactions of others and refuse to let people's actual or imagined responses to your stuttering continue to affect your mental health or your peace of mind.

This is easier said than done but it can be accomplished. I found that by facing my fears gradually I was able to achieve such a goal and I have known other stutterers who have "thrown" themselves into similar confrontations. Use whatever pace that best suits you but get involved, one way or another, in these confrontations with your "speech fears." There will be times when you will be unable to face the fears inherent in different situations, but persevere. Don't give up! Continue facing your fears as often as you can. Besides the peace of mind that develops, you will also become more fluent in your speech.   (Adler)

What kind of a job should a stutterer try to get?

On the whole, people who stutter are highly intelligent and capable. Yet there appears to be a discrepancy between their realistic capacities and potentialities and what they unrealistically expect of themselves. Although there are many areas of productivity through which an individual can express his capacities and earn a comfortable living, I have found that many stutterers seem to be drawn toward jobs or professions where the use of verbal communication is paramount. It is not uncommon to find people who have difficulty speaking attempting to become salesmen, lawyers, psychologists, and radio announcers. There is no serious objection to this endeavor provided stuttering does not interfere too greatly. As a stutterer you can become successful in most jobs or occupations.   (Barbara)

Why not substitute easier words?

You will feel better about your speech if you reduce the

number of times you substitute non-feared words for feared ones. To test this out make five telephone calls and keep an account of the number of times you substituted non-feared words for feared ones. Then make five more telephone calls in which you try to make as few substitutions as possible. You should feel better about your speech when you are not substituting words or switching phrases to avoid stuttering. You may find that your fear of stuttering is actually *more* of a problem than your stuttering. (Trotter)

Why not just avoid the problem?

Crucial to this point is the fact that struggle and avoidance *worsen* a problem of stuttering. Easy repetitions of sounds become hard repetitions with tension and facial contortion when force and hurry are added to them. Audiences react negatively to the struggle, and this convinces you that you must "try harder" so you increase your struggle. Similarly, penalty reactions to your stuttering prompt you to avoid or conceal your stuttering. Your speech becomes cautious and backward-moving. Your attention is directed to planning escape from stuttered words rather than to planning your thoughts. Avoidance strengthens your need to be fluent. The most evil part of his development is the subtle way in which struggle and avoidance become a part of you. They become involuntary and you do not recognize when you use them. (Moses)

———

Stuttering is an anticipatory, apprehensive, hypertonic avoidance reaction.

Your stuttering is simply the things you do trying to avoid what you think of as stuttering, and that there is no stuttering to avoid if you do nothing to avoid it. It leads you, therefore, to wonder why, after all, you should try to keep from doing something that you will not do anyway, if you didn't try to keep from doing it. (Johnson)

Determine to reduce your use of avoidances. Try to stutter openly and audibly. Let your stutterings be heard and seen rather than continue to conceal them by hurry and quiet. Try to keep your stuttering forward-moving and purposeful rather than postponed and half-hearted. Try to maintain eye contact with your listeners. Looking away severs the communication link with your audience and convinces them that you are ashamed and disgusted with the way that you talk. When you present yourself in an embarrassed and uncomfortable way you are more likely to receive negative audience reactions than if you stutter openly and severely. Deliberately enter previously feared situations. Judge your performance on the basis of the degree to which you approached the situation rather than on the basis of how much you stuttered or how fluent you were. Begin to recognize yourself as you are and as you want to be rather than as you think others want you to be. All of us need to be loved by, and in close contact with, other people. However, too much "human respect" makes us prisoners of what we think others want us to be. (Moses)

Above all, keep in mind that the less you struggle in your efforts not to stutter, and the less you avoid feared words and situations, the less you will stutter in the long run. (J. D. Williams)

In his efforts to speak fluently, the stutterer becomes more and more fearful of being unable to cope with the intermittent stuttering that may occur. The more he struggles to avoid possible stuttering or attempts to hide or disguise his stuttering that cannot be avoided, the more he denies that he has a problem. (Czuchna)

Is stuttering funny?

Most people are somewhat tense talking to stutterers because they do not know how to react. Perhaps they believe that the stutterer is very sensitive about his problem and are afraid they will say or do something that will hurt his feelings. One way to make your listener feel at ease about your stuttering is to tell an occasional joke about it. If you are in a bad block and just can't get the word out you might say, "Well, if I don't get this word out soon we might be here all night." It's a good idea to have a healthy sense of humor about your stuttering. You might try one or two of these jokes on your friends to see if it puts them a little more at ease when talking to you. (Trotter)

Perhaps the day shall come when I can completely forgive those who have ridiculed and imitated my stuttering. As yet I have failed to find any more excuse for this than laughing at the crippled or the blind. I believe that those who torment the stutterer do so to compensate for some weakness or shortcoming of their own. (Wedberg)

How can one introduce himself?

Between the ages of fifteen and twenty I worked rather intensely on my speech and gradually realized that I would need to work on situations of increasing difficulty by planning, experiencing and the planning again, etc., until I became more and more confident. For example, during my freshman year in college I worked on introducing myself. After working to keep eye contact with my listener, I worked on modifying my speech and using some voluntary disfluency when saying "I'm Hugo Gre-Gregory." By the end of the year I never avoided introducing myself or making introductions. (Gregory)

Is the stutterer inferior or neurotic?

Because you stutter, it doesn't mean that you are biologically inferior or more neurotic than the next person. Maybe a little fortification with that knowledge may help you to accept yourself as a stutterer or feel more comfortable and be open about it. (Sheehan)

Shouldn't one try to talk perfectly?

Normal speech contains disfluences of many types. (Moses)

It is good for you to realize that much of your own hesitating and fumbling in speaking is like that of other folks. If you are like other speakers who think of themselves as stutterers, you tend to suppose that unless your speech flows as smoothly as a meadow brook you are not talking normally. Actually, many of your disfluencies are like those of normal speakers and are so regarded by them when they hear you. (Johnson)

A perfect flow of language formulation and speech production is a rare skill. Most of us have errors in formulation and imperfections in our speech production. . . . Compare what you do with what your friends do. They also repeat sounds, words and phrases, interject "uh" or stop while saying a difficult word. Therapy should lead toward acceptable, free flowing speech but not *perfect fluency*. (Boehmler)

The stutterer has a Demosthenes* complex. He makes demands on his speech and intellect which are excessive and impossible to achieve. This verbal perfectionism creates inner chaos and turmoil. The person who tends toward stuttering feels that he should always speak calmly, *never* ap-

---

* Demosthenes lived in the fourth century B.C. and is considered one of the greatest orators of all time. He was such a powerful speaker that his orations rallied the citizens of Athens to oppose and defeat Alexander the Great, which significantly affected the history of ancient Greece. Supposedly, he overcame a speech defect (stuttering?) by standing on the seashore with pebbles under his tongue and shouting above the roar of the waves.

pear ruffled and *constantly* be in control of his listener. When he speaks he demands of himself the ultimate and impossible. He feels he should be the master of his words and have a reservoir of everflowing facts and ideas. He should speak in a clear and concise manner, pause at the right time, and never run ahead of his ideas and be continually spontaneous when talking. . . . To avoid this dilemma make your expectations more reasonable.   (Barbara)

Maybe Demosthenes had the right idea?

Growing up as a severe stutterer, I would hear such stories almost daily, starting with the legend of Demosthenes pebbles. After trying everything else, I did attempt to talk with pebbles myself once. I didn't quite believe the legend, but I felt I should leave no stones untried. I almost swallowed the pebbles and quickly resumed the search for new crutches.   (Gregory)

What kind of advice do you get?

Every stutterer grows up with the naive advice of neighbors and casual strangers ringing uselessly in his ears. "Relax, think what you have to say, slow down, take a deep breath, did you ever try to talk with pebbles in your mouth, etc. etc."

Stuttering is a complex problem whose nature forever tempts people to offer simplistic cures. Neighbors and casual acquaintances usually do not offer advice on treating cancer or diabetes. But stuttering has a persistence along with a now-you-see-it-now-you-don't quality, so it fosters irresponsible and/or fraudulent claims for every solution. Simplistic "cures" abound, and the history of medicine is littered with them. Even intelligent people who should know better are taken in, or ensnare themselves.   (Sheehan)

———

For years most adult stutterers have received well meaning suggestions that have been directly or indirectly aimed at stopping the stuttering altogether. These suggestions imply miraculously quick cures and fluent speech. "Take a deep breath before a word on which you may stutter, then say it without stuttering." "Think of what you're going to say before you say it, and you won't have any trouble" etc. (Czuchna)

Stuttering is also a disorder which can be worsened by ill treatment. Many well-meaning but ignorant individuals, by their suggestions and reactions, have made the stuttering not only more difficult to bear but also more severe and frequent. As in all speech disorders, this one needs special understanding. (VanRiper)

Shouldn't one pretend not to be a stutterer?

You've tried to cover up, to keep a pretense as a fluent speaker. You get tired of this phony role. . . . You probably don't realize how much your coverup and avoidance keeps you in the vicious circle of stuttering. (Sheehan)

––––––––

I learned long ago that the harder I tried to camouflage my stuttering, the more severely I stuttered. It was a vicious circle and I wanted out. So I got out! How? I stopped stuttering severely with much less effort than I once used in trying in the wrong way to stop. And the wrong ways were to try to run from it, hide from it and forget it. I made the mistake of using every trick in the book to pretend to be a normal speaker, but none of the tricks worked for long. Failures only increased, and after years of agony I finally discovered that it was finally time to make an about-face. Why try to avoid and camouflage stuttering any longer? Who was I trying to fool? I knew that I stuttered, and so did my listeners. I finally took time out to ask myself why I should continue to fight the old, destructive feelings in the wrong way. I began to look at those feelings, and as I began to accept them and my stuttering, success in speaking began. It is interesting that the old ways of struggling were so difficult to give up. It felt as though I had an angry tiger by the tail and dared not let go.   (Rainey)

Sometimes it is helpful to explain something about your stuttering to people who are important to you. This person might be a parent, teacher, friend, employer or a fellow worker. You might explain, for example, how you would like to be treated by your listener when you are stuttering. The purpose of this is to make you and the people you speak with more relaxed concerning your stuttering. If you feel that a person understands your stuttering you are likely to stutter less to that person. An open and honest attitude is healthy for all people involved.   (Trotter)

At about this time I began my training as a speech pathologist and embarked upon a career, as my wife and children tell friends, of being a "professional stutterer." By the way, I've always noticed that when my wife tells some person "Hugo is a professional stutterer," the person looks somewhat perplexed as if to say, "Does he stutter?" or, "Why do you mention it?" The point is that we are very open about my stuttering. I found out very early that this attitude is an important ingredient in therapy.   (Gregory)

Should one monitor his speech?

Your first job is to observe what you do continuously, a process you call "monitoring." If you really monitor well, you will begin to drop many of your crutches automatically. (Sheehan)

The stutterer must come to know just what he does when he approaches a feared word or situation.

You must be able to analyze your own stuttering in terms of its varying symptoms.   (VanRiper)

When you are openly tackling the majority of your moments of stuttering you can try to change their form. Look at your stutterings objectively rather than emotionally. Study them by holding on to them longer than it would have taken to stutter-out the troublesome word. Resist the impulse to get the stuttering over with quickly. Although it is difficult to become less emotional about what you do, you need to become more realistic about yourself. For awhile, you must place greater emphasis on recognizing how you talk rather than on what others think of you.   (Moses)

———

John was able to observe his talking in a mirror and listen to it on a tape recording in order to begin to ask questions about what he could do about it. He observed in detail the process of normal speaking. We sat and read together so he could observe the feeling and movement involved in talking. He then tried to duplicate the behavior involved in his stuttering behavior and to describe the difference between it and normal talking. I began to make assignments for him. These assignments were undertaken not to learn any "skill" but rather to make observations of his behavior - to learn from his own behavior. Basic to all this was the question of how one can change these ways of acting.   (D. Williams)

Can one change?

"The leopard can't change its spots." If you are in the habit of thinking and saying things like that, you are likely to tell yourself also "once a stutterer always a stutterer"— you might then go on to the depressing thought that there's really no hope for you.

Or if there is, there is the wishful hope that somewhere sometime you will be lucky and find someone who will take away, or drive away, what you *have* and transform you, as though by sorcery, from the stutterer you are into the normal speaker you long to be one day.

Such wishfulness makes for dreams, particularly day-dreams, about magical potions in the form of pills, or secret or mysterious methods that can work wonders. It does not encourage you to face up to the problem yourself and do something constructive about it here and now by your own efforts.

What you have learned to do that keeps you from speaking better than you do, you can unlearn.   (Johnson)

———

Putting stuttering in a more realistic perspective may reduce some of your tension and make it easier for you to work on it.   (Luper)

Does recovery take long?

Recovery is going to be a long gradual process. (Murray)

———

If the stutterer is going to change radically his accustomed manner of stuttering, he must work persistently and diligently over a long period of time.   (Johnson)

———

When you go into therapy, when you begin to modify your speech pattern, go full tilt, reach for the home run. . . . Quit feeling sorry for yourself.   (Emerick)

A memorable experience

One score and seven years ago, in a desperate attempt to cure their son's chronic speech problem, my parents spent their meagre savings to send me to a commercial school for stammering. Alas, to their dismay and my deepening feeling of hopelessness, it was just another futile attempt. While I rode woefully toward home on the train, a kindly old gray-haired conductor stopped at my seat and asked my destination. I opened my mouth for the well-rehearsed "Detroit" but all that emerged was a series of muted gurgles; I pulled my abdominal muscles in hard to break the terrifying constriction in my throat—silence. Finally, the old man peered at me through his bifocals, shook his head and, with just the trace of a smile, said, "Well, young man, either express yourself or go by freight."

The conductor had shuffled on down the aisle of the rocking passenger car before the shock waves swept over me. Looking out the window at the speeding landscape through a tearful mist of anger and frustration, I felt the surreptitious glances of passengers seated nearby; a flush of crimson embarrassment crept slowly up my neck and my head throbbed with despair. Long afterwards I remembered the conductor's penetrating comment. For years I licked that and other stuttering wounds and nursed my wrath to keep it warm, dreaming that someday I would right all those unrightable wrongs. But in the end his pithy pun changed my life. The old man, incredibly, had been right.   (Emerick)

Boyhood recollections

What I remember most acutely about my stuttering is not the strangled sound of my own voice but the impatient looks on other people's faces when I had trouble getting a word out. And if their eyes happened to reflect some of the pain and frustration I was feeling, that only made me more uneasy. There was nothing they could do to help me, and I certainly didn't want their sympathy. I was nine or ten at the time.

Like most people with a stuttering problem, I had already learned to live by my wits in a way that normally fluent people cannot begin to appreciate. Whenever I opened my mouth, I mentally glanced ahead at the sentence I wanted to say, to see if there was any word I was likely to stutter on.

For me, speaking was like riding down a highway and

reading aloud from a series of billboards. I knew that to speak normally I had to keep moving forward at a steady pace. Yet every once in a while I became aware of an obstacle, like an enormous boulder, blocking the road some five or six billboards ahead of me. I knew that when I got to that particular word I would be unable to say it. I never figured out why I stuttered on one word rather than another.

Some sounds—like the "m" sound at the beginning of a word—were particularly troublesome; but, even with these, the context was all-important. A sentence might have two words beginning with "m," such as "I'll have to ask my mother." The moment I framed this sentence in my mind, I knew that I would have no trouble pronouncing "my" but that "mother" would be impossible. My usual strategy at such times was to speed up and try to crash through the obstacle. When I succeeded, the sentence came out like this: "I'll [pause for deep breath] havetoaskmymother."

This trick worked just often enough to convince some people that I stuttered because I talked too fast. But when it failed I found myself struck dumb in midsentence, unable to go forward or turn back. There were times when I got as far as the first sound in the difficult word and could do nothing but repeat it like a broken record, in the classic stutter that is imitated—usually for laughs—in books and movies. More often, I had a complete block; I would try to form the first sound in the word and something inside me would snap shut, so that if I opened my mouth nothing came out.

At that point, I usually backed up and looked for a detour. Sometimes all I had to do was find a less troublesome word that meant the same thing. For example, I might be able to get away with something like "I'll have to check with my folks." If I couldn't think of a synonym quickly enough, I had no choice but to rephrase the sentence, to try to sneak up on the difficult word from another direction; the result might come out as: "You know how mothers are, I better ask her first."

I didn't have the slightest idea why the same word should be easier to say in one context than in another, but whenever it worked out that way I felt absurd pride in my accomplishment; no one else knew that in order to speak with any fluency I had to become a kind of walking thesaurus. But the strategies of substitution and circumlocution created their own problems. The farther I strayed from the original wording of the sentence, the more I had to guard against letting subtle changes of meaning creep in.

If I wasn't careful, I could find myself saying things I didn't quite mean, just to be able to say something. In a way, my situation was not so different from that of a writer in a totalitarian country who tries to communicate under the constant threat of censorship. The fact that I carried the censor around inside my head did not make the situation any less oppressive.

(This last quotation comes from the book "Stuttering, The Disorder of Many Theories" by Gerald Jonas, published by Farrar, Straus & Giroux.)

Authors of Quotations

SOL ADLER, Ph.D.
Professor of Speech Pathology
University of Tennessee
Knoxville

JOSEPH G. AGNELLO, Ph.D.
Professor of Speech Pathology
University of Cincinnati

JAMES T. ATEN, Ph.D.
Chairman of Speech Pathology Section
V.A. Hospital, Long Beach, California

DOMINICK A. BARBARA, Ph.D., M.D.
Psychiatrist
Karen Horney Clinic, New York City

C. S. BLUEMEL, M.D.
*Late Fellow of the American
Psychiatric Association and the
American College of Physicians*

RICHARD M. BOEHMLER, Ph.D.
Professor of Speech Pathology
University of Montana, Missoula

JOHN L. BOLAND, Ph.D.
Clinical Psychiatrist
Oklahoma Psychological and
Educational Center
Oklahoma City

SPENCER F. BROWN, Ph.D., M.D.
formerly Associate Professor of Pediatrics
University of Iowa

PAUL R. CZUCHNA, M.A.
Director of Stuttering Programs
Western Michigan University, Kalamazoo

LON L. EMERICK, Ph.D.
Professor of Speech Pathology
Northern Michigan University, Marquette

HENRY FREUND, M.D.
Fellow American Psychiatric Association
Milwaukee, Wisconsin

HUGO L. GREGORY, Ph.D.
Professor of Speech Pathology
Northwestern University
Evanston, Illinois

WENDELL JOHNSON, Ph.D.
formerly Professor of Speech Pathology
and Director of Speech Clinic
University of Iowa

GARY N. LaPORTE, M.A.
formerly Coordinator of
Speech Pathology Programs
University of Tampa

HAROLD L. LUPER, Ph.D.
Professor and Head, Speech
Pathology Department
University of Tennessee, Knoxville

FREDERICK MARTIN, M.D.
formerly Superintendent of
Speech Corrections
New York City Schools

GERALD R. MOSES, Ph.D.
Associate Professor of Speech Pathology
Eastern Michigan University
Ypsilanti

FREDERICK P. MURRAY, Ph.D.
Director, Division of Speech Pathology
University of New Hampshire, Durham

MARGARET M. NEELY, Ph.D.
Director, Baton Rouge Speech
and Hearing Foundation
Louisiana

MARGARET RAINEY, Ph.D.
Director, Speech Pathology
Shorewood Public Schools, Wisconsin

JOSEPH G. SHEEHAN, Ph.D.
Professor of Psychology
University of California, Los Angeles

HAROLD B. STARBUCK, Ph.D.
Professor of Speech Pathology
State University of New York, Geneseo

COURTNEY STROMSTA, Ph.D.
Professor of Speech Pathology
Western Michigan University
Kalamazoo

WILLIAM D. TROTTER, Ph.D.
Director, Communicative Disorders
Marquette University, Milwaukee

CHARLES VANRIPER, Ph.D.
*Distinguished Professor Emeritus of
Speech Pathology*
Western Michigan University
Kalamazoo

CONRAD WEDBERG, M.A.
formerly Director of Speech Therapy
Alhambra City School, California

DEAN WILLIAMS, Ph.D.
Professor of Speech Pathology
University of Iowa, Iowa City

J. DAVID WILLIAMS, Ph.D.
Professor of Speech Pathology
Northern Illinois University, DeKalb

All quotations are from published writings including the following books: A Clinician's Guide to Stuttering; Sol Adler (Charles C. Thomas). Questions and Answers on Stuttering; Dominick A. Barbara (Charles C. Thomas). The Psychotherapy of Stuttering; Dominick A. Barbara, Ed. (Charles C. Thomas). The Riddle of Stuttering; C. S. Bluemel (Interstate Publishing). Stuttering, A Second Symposium; Jon Eisenson, Ed. (Harper & Row). An Analysis of Stuttering; Emerick and Hamre, Ed. (Interstate Publishers). Psychopathology and the Problems of Stuttering; Henry Freund (Charles C. Thomas). Controversies About Stuttering Therapy; Hugo Gregory, Ed. (University Park Press). Learning Theory and Stuttering Therapy; Hugo Gregory, Ed. (Northwestern University Press). People in Quandaries; Wendell Johnson (Harper & Brothers). Speech Handicapped School Children; Wendell Johnson, Ed. (Harper & Brothers). Stuttering in Children and Adults; Wendell Johnson, Ed. (Harper & Brothers). Stuttering and What You Can Do About It; Wendell Johnson (University of Minnesota Press). Speech Problems of Children; Wendell Johnson, Ed. (Grune & Stratton). Stuttering, Research and Therapy; Joseph Sheehan, Ed. (Harper & Brothers). Handbook of Speech Pathology; Lee Edward Travis, Ed. (Appleton-Century-Crofts). Speech Correction; Charles VanRiper (Prentice-Hall). The Nature of Stuttering; Charles Van Riper (Prentice-Hall). The Treatment of Stuttering; Charles VanRiper (Prentice-Hall). Speech Therapy, A Book of Readings; Charles VanRiper, Ed. (Prentice-Hall). The Stutterer Speaks; Conrad Wedberg (Expression Co.), and from the publications of the Speech Foundation of America.

Glossary

Many speech pathology words or terms are listed in this glossary which are not used in the book. These are inserted for the information or education of those readers who may not be familiar with the meanings of expressions frequently used in books and articles about the therapy of stuttering, including some relating to the prevention of stuttering in very young children.

---

anticipatory reactions. The abnormal actions or movements exhibited by a stutterer when approaching a feared word; the speaking behavior of the stutterer in his attempts to try to avoid the difficulty he is expecting; feelings experienced and behavior exhibited before the overt performance of stuttering.

anxiety. In stuttering a state of apprehension or fear often pertaining to anticipations of unsatisfactory or disrupting interpersonal relationships, such as anticipation of 'difficulty' when speaking. This state of anxiety may be an integral element in the stutterer's fear of verbal difficulty.

articulation. Literally, a joining; in speech the utterance of the individual sounds of speech in connected discourse; the movements during speech of the organs that modify the stream of voiced and unvoiced breath in meaningful sounds: the speech function performed largely through movements of the mandible, lips, tongue and soft palate.

auditory feedback. The sensations produced by stimulation of the ear by one's own speech, either by air-borne or bone-conducted vibrations—to be distinguished from the tactile, kinesthetic, and possibly visual (as in a mirror) sensations which also result from speech.

avoidance. The action(s) the stutterer makes in trying to dodge stuttering or in endeavoring to avoid trouble talking. Consists of postponements, stallers, retrials, use of synonyms, circumlocutions, etc.

block (or blocking). A moment of stuttering; stuttering behavior; a unit of nonfluency; refers to the stuttering behavior that happens at the instant the speech muscles do not function normally; or to the stoppage or obstruction experienced by the stutterer in trying to talk, temporarily preventing smooth progress.

bounce. The voluntary repetition several times of the first sound or syllable of a word in an easy, effortless fashion.

cluttering. Excessively rapid talking in which syllables or words are omitted or repeated and the articulation is slurred or jumbled. The tempo of the speech is generally jerky and word groups are spoken in rapid spurts, making the speech difficult to understand. This disorder is frequently confused with stuttering. The clutterer, unlike the stutterer, can usually speak normally when he speaks slowly and carefully.

conditioning. Often used as a synonym for any kind of learning; but more specifically refers to any of several procedures (see 'operant conditioning') in which one arranges for certain stimuli to occur at an appropriate time so that a particular response is made to occur either more often (acquisition) or less often (extinction). When a response that formerly occurred only rarely or not at all is 'conditioned' to occur more often, learning is assumed to have taken place, provided that the change is long-lasting. It is theorized by some pathologists that all learning is a result of conditioning processes that take place either by chance or through the conscious manipulation of stimuli by others.

consonant. A conventional speech sound characterized by constriction or closure at one or more points in the breath channel; broadly, any sound in a syllable other than the vowel sound.

delayed auditory feedback. The hearing by a speaker of his own utterance after a brief time interval; in laboratory applications the delay is usually of the order of 0.1 or 0.2 second; in an echo effect sometimes observed in a valley or a football stadium, for example, the delay may be as long as a second or more. This delayed auditory feedback, usually artificially created by a mechanical device, slows and disrupts the speech of many speakers. Sometimes used with the stutterer to establish a slow, prolonged pattern of speech (emphasizing proprioceptive control), which the stutterer must adopt to overcome the disruptive or punishing effects of the delayed auditory feedback.

desensitization. The process of toughening of a person to the stress in certain situations by increasing the person's ability to confront his problem with less anxiety, guilt or hostility.

developmental hesitations. The normal repetitions, prolongations or stumblings in the speech of a child learning to talk. In the natural development of speech, while learning to talk, most children's speech is marked by effortless developmental hesitations to a greater or lesser extent. Includes word and phrase repetitions and such accessory vocalizations as "um" and "uh."

diagnosogenic theory. The theory, set forth by Wendell Johnson, that "stuttering as a clinical problem, as a definite disorder, was found to occur not before being diagnosed but *after being diagnosed.*" According to this theory, the problem of stuttering arises when a listener, usually a parent, evaluates or classifies or diagnoses the child's developmental hesitations and repetitions as stuttering, and reacts to them as a consequence with concern and disapproval, and as the child senses this concern and disapproval he reacts by speaking more hesitantly and with concern of his own, and finally with the tensing and struggle involved in the effort to keep from hesitating or repeating.

differential relaxation. The lessening of tension by the stutterer of one set of muscles connected with the production of speech regardless of how tense other muscles may be.

disfluency or **dysfluency.** Refers to any kind of speech which is not smooth or fluent. All speakers talk disfluently at times, i.e. they hesitate or stumble in varying degree. All stutterers are disfluent but all disfluency is not stuttering. For instance 'disfluency' could describe the developmental hesitations of a child learning to talk or the arrhythmic breaks in the speech of an adult, etc. Some therapists use the term 'nonfluency'.

distraction. Diversion of the attention; filling the mind with other thoughts so that the expectancy of stuttering is kept out; keeping the anticipation of stuttering from consciousness, thus temporarily effecting release from fear of stuttering and the performance of stuttering reactions.

eye contact. Looking the listener in the eye while talking to him. Generally a natural, although not a constant, interaction of the speaker's eyes with the eyes of the listener.

fear. Is to the stutterer the apprehension of unpleasantness which arises when he consciously perceives situations which lead him to anticipate difficulty in talking. This fear of difficulty may be and often is intense. It can and sometimes does temporarily paralyze thought and action. Stuttering is usually relatively proportionate to the amount of such fear present. Stuttering fears may be of situations or persons, of sounds or words, of the telephone, etc.

feared word. This term refers to a word, or one of its sounds on which the stutterer anticipates difficulty.

feedback. The reinforcing effects of the stutterer's auditory or proprioceptive perception of his own speech. Technically the partial return of the effects of a process to its source so as to reinforce, reduce, or otherwise modify it.

fixation(s). The maintenance of an articulatory or phonatory posture for an abnormal duration; the arresting of the speech muscles in a rigid position temporarily blocking speech, a variety of stuttering behavior.

frustration tolerance. The capacity of the stutterer to resist feelings of frustration because of his inability to speak without difficulty; the ability to put up with or endure the communication handicaps resulting from not being able to talk freely.

group therapy. The counseling of and among stutterers in a group, including the use of speech within such social situations. The interchange of feelings, ideas and discussions about stuttering problems in a group gives the stutterer emotional release and helps him to develop better insight and understanding through a knowledge of how others react to their problems.

hypnotism. A state of behavior induced by a hypnotist. When hypnotized a stutterer may speak freely or more fluently than he can in his ordinary state of awareness. However, it has not been shown that suggestions made during hypnosis have any permanent effect on the stutterer's ordinary speech behavior.

hysterical stuttering. Stuttering, usually temporary, resulting from acute excitement or the result of shock or neurotic need.

in-block correction. See Page 97.

inhibition. Restraint on one's ability to act by either conscious or subconscious processes; the partial checking or complete blocking of one impulse or mental process by another nearly simultaneous impulse or mental process. The fear of stuttering tends to inhibit the stutterer's impulse or desire to speak.

learned behavior. Any relatively permanent change in a person's behavior resulting from his reaction to or interaction with environmental influences or from reinforced practice; an acquired neuro-muscular, verbal, emotional, or other type of response to certain stimuli.

light contacts. Loose or non-tensed contacts of the lips and/or tongue on plosive sounds. Contacts of the lips and/or tongue which are optimal for the production of speech sounds as contrasted to the hard, tense contacts which are often a part of the stuttering pattern.

mirror observation practice. Self analysis through mirror study; practicing reading or speaking in front of a mirror so that the stutterer can observe his stuttering reactions so as to study ways of modifying or eliminating them.

modifying the stuttering pattern. Refers to the stutterer changing what he does when he stutters. Clinicians suggest that he can and should deliberately change his stuttering behavior and learn to stutter in different ways and usually in an easier manner. In so modifying his stuttering pattern he learns that he can change his way of speaking and that he can develop a style of talking which is less abnormal and free of excessive tensing.

monitoring. A technique in which the stutterer seeks to become highly aware of the articulatory movements of his speech, as well as other behaviors, which make up his characteristic and habitual pattern of stuttering. This would include continuous self-observation of the crutches and tricks he uses in his act of stuttering.

nonfluency. Refers to speech which is not smooth or fluent. All speakers talk nonfluently at times, i.e. they hesitate or stumble in varying degree. All stutterers are nonfluent but all nonfluency is not stuttering. For instance 'nonfluency' could be used to describe the developmental hesitations of a child learning to talk or the arrhythmic breaks in the normal speech of an adult, etc. Same as 'disfluency.'

objective attitude. Referring to the attitude that it is desirable for the stutterer to have toward his stuttering; a feeling relatively independent of one's personal prejudices or apprehensions and not distorted by shame or embarrassment; the acceptance of his stuttering as a problem rather than a curse.

operant conditioning. A method by which a response to a stimulus may be learned by controlling its consequences through reinforcement; any of a variety of procedures in which the experimenter or the clinician arranges for a stimulus to occur following the occurrence of a response. If the stimulus is a pleasant one, the response it follows will occur more often, but if the stimulus is a disagreeable one, the response it follows will occur less often. This process is often theorized to be the way in which voluntary behaviors are learned. Behaviorists consider this as the basic strategy for achieving behavior change. According to the basic principle of operant conditioning, stuttering behavior will occur more or less depending on the consequences it generates.

oscillation(s). In stuttering the tremorous vibrations or repetitions of speech muscle movements temporarily blocking speech; often used with 'fixation(s)'—see that word.

parent counseling. Involves establishing a personalized relationship between the parent and a therapist to enable the latter to influence the home environment and particularly the feelings, habits, and policies of the parents as regards the child, so as to diminish anxiety-provoking environmental conditions as much as possible. Since parental attitudes can be the cause or part of the cause of a child's stuttering and a healthy emotional atmosphere in the home is desirable in stuttering therapy, wise and effective parental counseling is important.[1]

[1]*First:* Make no issue of your child's repetitions and hesitations in speaking. *Second:* Eliminate or modify any conditions that tend to make your child speak with unusual amounts or kinds of repetitions and hesitations. *Third:* Do everything you can to make speaking rewarding or fun for your child. *Fourth:* Do everything you can to be a good listener for your child. *Fifth:* Do everything you can to make speech a personal sharing for you and your child. (Wendell Johnson)

phonation. Vocalization; act or process of uttering voice; production of the voiced sounds of speech.

plosive. As a noun, any speech sound made by impounding the air stream momentarily until pressure has been developed and then suddenly releasing it, as in 'p' 'b' 't' 'd' 'k' or 'q'. As an adjective, designating the characteristic of a plosive, especially that phase in which the air is held for a moment under pressure.

post-block correction. See Page 85.

postponement devices. Stutterers frequently respond to the perception of impending difficulty in the utterance of a word by pausing before attempting it. To disguise this pause, they often use other words or sounds or retrials of previously spoken words.

pre-block correction. See Page 91.

progressive relaxation. A technique for teaching an awareness of the state of tension in muscle groups throughout the body and an ability to bring about decreased tension when under stress. Some clinicians make use of this procedure to accomplish various objectives in stuttering therapy.

prolongation. The lengthening in time, or prolonging, of a speech sound or posture of the lips, tongue, or other parts of the speech mechanism, or a fricative such as the sound of the letter *s*; the stutterer may say "a—pple," prolonging the 'a' in apple, or he may say "b—a—by" for example, or "mmmother". Easy prolongation of the vowel sound on both feared and nonfeared words is used quite extensively to modify the stuttering pattern. See 'modifying the stuttering pattern'.

proprioception. A general term used to cover both kinesthesia (the awareness of bodily movement and position) and taction (the sense of touch or contact). Speech apparently is monitored both through auditory and through proprioceptive feedback.

psychoneurosis. A nervous disorder or an emotional maladjustment which results in or involves deviate behavior; an abnormality of the personality structure which is a disguised reaction to some psychic irritant. In the medical field the theory is widely held that stuttering is a symptom of a psychoneurotic condition, but most speech pathologists appear to reject largely or wholly the view that stuttering is a psychoneurosis.

psychotherapy. The treatment of behavioral or emotional problems, such as stuttering, by counseling, or by re-education and influencing the person's mental approaches and his ways of thinking, or of evaluating his problems; any procedures intended to improve the condition of a person that are directed at a change in his mental approach to his problems, particularly his attitude toward himself and his environment.

Don't expect that psychotherapy will help your stuttering much. A psychiatrist or psychologist is trained to deal with emotional or neurotic problems. (Brown)

pull-out. Based on the hypothesis that it is possible for a stutterer to pull out of difficulty during a block, this term refers to a voluntarily controlled release from the stuttering block. (See "in-block correction".)

rate control. A technique in which the stutterer attempts to speak more slowly, often in a monotone with each syllable given equal stress, possibly in a chanting sing-song style.

regression. Having more speech difficulty usually as a result of reverting back to an earlier faulty manner of talking.

resonant. Having a pleasantly loud full quality, low pitched voice. Speaking with vocalizations that are fully relaxed, adequately loud and appropriately long.

secondary symptoms. The abnormal actions or movements exhibited by a stutterer in trying to talk. These include, but are not limited to eye blinks, arm swinging, grimaces, head or body jerks, foot stompings, clearing the throat, excessive use of 'uhs' or 'wells'. Actually *any* ways by which the stutterer characteristically and abnormally approaches a feared word or struggles to release himself from a movement of verbal inability.

slide. Uttering the different sounds of a syllable in transitory slow motion often with prolongation of the vowel; sliding through a syllable on which stuttering is anticipated.

speech pathology. The science or study of disorders of speech, language and voice and their diagnosis and treatment.

stammering. Synonymous with 'stuttering'.

starter. Refers to any means or device which the stutterer has acquired as a means of 'breaking' a block in order to start the words he intends to say. These reactions can be any unnatural movement such as eye blinking, arm swinging, head jerking, clearing the throat, excessive use of "uhs," "wells," etc. This word recalls the popular notion that to "whistle" may help a person to say a word on which he is 'stuck.'

stuttering. Stuttering is a communication disorder characterized by excessive involuntary disruptions or blockings in the flow of speech, particularly when such disruptions consist of repetitions or prolongations of a sound or syllable, and when they are accompanied by avoidance struggle behavior.

Note: Most speech pathologists frown on labeling the developmental hesitations of a child learning to talk as 'stuttering' when there are no avoidance or struggle reactions.

stuttering pattern. In the case of the individual stutterer, refers to the particular way he experiences difficulty in talking, or the specific things he does, and the order in which he does these things that interfere with his speaking; the particular sequence of reactions in his stuttering speech behavior.

therapist, speech. A person professionally trained in the treatment of speech disorders. Also referred to as speech clinician, speech correctionist, remedial speech specialist, speech consultant, speech pathologist or logopedist.

therapy. The treatment of any clinically significant condition, such as stuttering; a program or method of instruction, supervised practice or counseling.

time pressure. At the moment the stutterer is expected to speak he often has an almost panicky feeling of haste or urgency. He feels he is under 'time pressure' and with no time to lose, and so he has a somewhat compulsive feeling that he must speak instantly without allowing time for deliberate and relaxed expression.

tremor. Tiny vibrations of the lips or jaw.

voluntary stuttering. In speech therapy refers to a manner of talking in which the stutterer in a conscious way imitates a pattern of stuttering. Voluntary stuttering may take the form of easy prolongation, or relatively spontaneous and effortless repetition, of the first sound or syllable of a word or the word itself. This style of talking may be used as a deliberate replacement for the usual stuttering behavior and it is intended to reduce fear of difficulty by voluntary doing that which is dreaded. This conscious affectation of repetitions (or other forms of disfluency, including prolongations, hesitations, etc.) is also designed to eliminate other avoidance reactions.

vowel. A voiced speech sound in the articulation of which the oral part of the breath channel is not blocked and not constricted enough to cause audible friction; broadly, the most prominent sound in a syllable.

*If you feel that this book has helped you
and you wish to help the cause,
send a donation to*

Speech Foundation of America
152 Lombardy Road,
Memphis, Tennessee 38111.
Contributions are tax deductible.

The Speech Foundation of America
is a non-profit charitable organization
dedicated to the prevention and therapy
of stuttering.

Publication Number 11

IF YOUR CHILD STUTTERS:
A GUIDE FOR PARENTS

An interesting, understandable and authoritative book for parents of young children three to six years of age. It describes and explains what they can and should do to prevent their child from developing into a confirmed stutterer—a 48-page book—50¢.

Available from

THE SPEECH FOUNDATION OF AMERICA
152 Lombardy Road
Memphis, Tenn. 38111